Valuing Health

Valuing Health

The Generalized and Risk-Adjusted
Cost-Effectiveness (GRACE) Model

CHARLES E. PHELPS

AND

DARIUS N. LAKDAWALLA

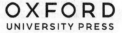

OXFORD
UNIVERSITY PRESS

OXFORD
UNIVERSITY PRESS

Oxford University Press is a department of the University of Oxford. It furthers
the University's objective of excellence in research, scholarship, and education
by publishing worldwide. Oxford is a registered trade mark of Oxford University
Press in the UK and certain other countries.

Published in the United States of America by Oxford University Press
198 Madison Avenue, New York, NY 10016, United States of America.

Library of Congress Cataloging-in-Publication Data
Names: Phelps, Charles E., author. | Lakdawalla, Darius N.
Title: Valuing health : the generalized and risk-adjusted cost-effectiveness
(GRACE) model / Charles E. Phelps and Darius N. Lakdawalla.
Description: New York, NY : Oxford University Press, [2024] |
Includes bibliographical references and index. |
Identifiers: LCCN 2023017324 (print) | LCCN 2023017325 (ebook) |
ISBN 9780197686294 (paperback) | ISBN 9780197686287 (hardback) |
ISBN 9780197686317 (epub) | ISBN 9780197686324 (online)
Subjects: MESH: Cost-Effectiveness Analysis | Value-Based Health Care |
Health Policy—economics | Cost-Benefit Analysis | Quality of Life | United States
Classification: LCC RA410.53 (print) | LCC RA410.53 (ebook) |
NLM W 74 AA1 | DDC 338.4/73621—dc23/eng/20230505
LC record available at https://lccn.loc.gov/2023017324
LC ebook record available at https://lccn.loc.gov/2023017325

DOI: 10.1093/oso/9780197686287.001.0001

Paperback printed by Marquis Book Printing, Canada
Hardback printed by Bridgeport National Bindery, Inc., United States of America

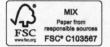

MIX
Paper from
responsible sources
FSC® C103567

To Dale and Emily,
Their value to us remains beyond measure.

CONTENTS

12. Welfare and Equity Implications of GRACE 217

13. Conclusions and Next Steps 241

A person who never made a mistake never tried anything new.

—ALBERT EINSTEIN

Cost-effectiveness analysis (CEA) has become the mainstay of many health care systems to estimate the value of medical interventions, and it is used at least as a reference point in many more. The subject is taught widely in graduate programs involving health care, such as Master of Public Health and Master of Public Policy, and in courses in medical schools and graduate business schools. It is also taught extensively through on-line and in-person courses from organizations such as the Society for Medical Decision Making and ISPOR—The International Society for Pharmacoeconomics and Outcomes Research, which has approximately 15,000 worldwide members. The Tufts University registry of CEA studies now contains more than 11,000 entries.[1] Clearly, CEA is a large and active "industry."

Many biopharmaceutical and medical device companies also have strong interests and capabilities in the conduct of health economics and outcomes research (HEOR), in part evidenced by substantial individual and organizational membership in such organizations as ISPOR and widespread participation in published economic evaluations of medical interventions.

The message of this book is that the basic model of value currently used in these studies is incomplete. Because of a simple (and almost certainly incorrect) assumption—that people do not have diminishing returns to health in producing utility—current models fail to capture important aspects of the value of medical interventions.

This omission leads to five systematic errors that distort health care resource allocation:

1. The willingness to pay (WTP) for low-illness-severity medical care is overstated.
2. The WTP for high-severity illnesses is correspondingly understated.
3. Alongside the errors in characterizing value for the severely ill, the existing model fails to characterize how permanent disability can increase the value of health improvements. In so doing, it understates the value of medical treatment for people with disabilities. The existing model states that improving the health of disabled people always has *less* value than for otherwise-comparable nondisabled people. This feature of the current model has led to a ban of its use for U.S. federal government decision-making about health care.
4. The current model ignores variability in treatment outcomes, assessing only mean differences in outcomes. When people experience diminishing returns to health, they also will dislike uncertain treatment outcomes, so ignoring this uncertainty can be misleading, especially when competing technologies have very similar mean gains in health outcomes.
5. The current model ignores how people with lower health-related quality of life (HRQoL) might have different preferences around trading life expectancy (LE) for improved HRQoL than people with higher HRQoL. Economic intuition suggests that a person in a very poor HRQoL state would be more willing to give up some LE in exchange for more HRQoL, but the current framework cannot accommodate this variability in preferences.

Why do we believe that diminishing returns to health are important? Think about the following questions outside the realm of health care:

Housing: Consider two people who are otherwise identical, one living in a small house with 1,200 square feet of space, the other living in a McMansion with 5,000 square feet of space. Which of these would gain more value with the addition of another 500 square feet of housing space?

Income: Consider two people who are otherwise identical, one with an annual income of $30,000, and the other with an annual income of $150,000. Now consider adding $10,000 to the annual income of each of these. To which of them would it bring greater added value?

Labor/leisure: Consider two otherwise identical people who hold jobs paying the same income, providing the same health insurance (and related) benefits, and providing the same on-job "ambience" at the workplace. Suppose one of these two jobs has 1 week of paid vacation each year, and the other has 4 weeks of annual paid vacation. To which would an additional week of paid vacation provide the greatest value?

In all these cases, economic models typically assume that for income, leisure, and other goods, adding the same additional amount of an economic "good" creates more added well-being (utility) when someone has less of that good to start with. This axiom of economic theory produces a number of implications that have passed empirical test after empirical test. From what we can tell, diminishing returns exist "everywhere." These cases all hinge on the concept of "scarcity," the relative shortage of some "good." Scarcity matters!

Of note, the presence of diminishing returns to income makes people averse to risks over their income, and the same is true for other goods. The widespread demand among consumers for insurance of all kinds testifies to their risk aversion regarding "money" (their ability to consume market goods and services) and thus to their diminishing returns as well. The provision of insurance, which can be dated at least back to the Code of Hammurabi in 1750 BCE in Babylon, testifies to the permanence of this phenomenon.

Yet, the theory of cost-effectiveness departs from this widespread approach. In the realm of health and well-being, we often use a HRQoL scale where 0 represents the worst imaginable health and 1 represents the best imaginable ("perfect") health. How do these ideas apply when involving people's health?

Start with a simple introspective question: Would you rather have a 1-hour massage if you were feeling "great" or if you had some strained muscles in your back? The latter condition has a lower HRQoL rating. If you said "when I have some strained muscles," then you are exhibiting diminishing returns to HRQoL.

Suppose there are two otherwise identical people, but one has a medical disorder such as a peptic ulcer, stress urinary incontinence, or benign prostatic hypertrophy, each of which are estimated to reduce HRQoL by approximately 0.1 on a scale of 0 to 1, a 10 percent loss per year. The other individual has secondary progressive multiple sclerosis, which is estimated to reduce HRQoL by approximately 0.6, a 60 percent loss per year. Which of these two people will gain greater value from a 0.1 per year HRQoL improvement?

A number of population surveys have addressed similar questions in detail. These studies typically conclude that HRQoL improvement is worth more to the patients in lower HRQoL states. Yet, traditional CEA assumes that such gains are worth the same, regardless of baseline HRQoL. Referring to the standard CEA summary of health gains, the Quality-Adjusted Life Year (QALY), the common mantra for CEA says that "a QALY is a QALY is a QALY." This assumption places cost-effectiveness out of step with the rest of economics and with the empirical evidence on how real people value health improvements.

Traditional CEA models imply that improving the health of a disabled person has less value than the same improvement for a nondisabled person. This has led the U.S. Affordable Care Act to forbid the use of any models to measure value of health care that "discount the value of life of a disabled person." Several attempts to remedy this problem assume counterfactual situations—for example, that disabled people are not in fact disabled (Nord et al., 1999; Basu et al., 2020). To us, this is an attempt to paper over the flaws in the underlying model. The problem with the traditional model is not how many QALYs disabled people have or gain but, rather, how they are valued, so "fixing" it by modifying the QALYs gained, we believe, is the wrong solution.

Proponents of standard CEA models defend its use by stating that nobody has ever really been denied medical care because of their disability status. This is clearly wrong, both indirectly and directly.

Indirectly, current methods send economic signals to developers of new technologies about what society values. This necessarily alters what levels of WTP will exist for new treatments that improve the well-being of persons with permanent disabilities. Therefore, incentives to develop cures for such disabilities are also altered.

Directly, before the Americans with Disabilities Act, many medical and dental clinics, lacking elevators, had stairsteps into their facilities that denied access to persons in wheelchairs or who had otherwise limited mobility. Even today, persistent barriers to care exist that could be, but have not been, remedied. The Center for Medicare and Medicaid Services has a major section in its Office of Minority Health to improve access for persons with disabilities.[2] Such a center would not exist if the problem itself did not exist.

A survey of U.S. physicians revealed that the problem indeed persists (Iezzoni et al., 2021). Although 82 percent of surveyed physicians believed that people with significant disability have worse HRQoL, less than half of those were confident that they could provide the same quality of care to disabled people as they provide to nondisabled people. Importantly, barely more than half of the surveyed doctors said that they would strongly welcome disabled patients into their practice.

The reasons for this can be complex, but one obvious issue stands out: The complications of accommodating patients' disabilities can be costly, and the health care reimbursement system does not readily recognize the value of paying for these added costs. Willingness to pay more for improving the HRQoL for disabled people is important, even though current CEA methods state that it is worth less, not more, to improve the health of disabled people. Our new approach shows why higher valuations exist for treating people with permanent disabilities, not just in the creation of new technologies but also in the day-to-day operation of the health care system.

We call our new approach the generalized risk-adjusted cost-effectiveness (GRACE) model. GRACE introduces declining returns to health into the value model, an assumption that is not only standard in the field of health economics but also parallels a vast literature in the economics of consumer behavior.[3] In so doing, it provides formal methods, based in rigorous economic theory, that demonstrate the following:

- Current methods overvalue the treatment of minor illnesses.
- Value per unit of health improvement often rises exponentially with the degree of illness severity, increasingly so as risk aversion in health rises.
- Improving HRQoL of disabled people is *more valuable*, not less valuable, compared with improving the health of otherwise similar nondisabled individuals.
- Treatments with less uncertain outcomes often have more value than otherwise similar treatments—for example, those with the same mean improvement in health outcomes. GRACE provides a precise way to measure those value differences, which we call "the value of insurance." Similarly, increased positive skewness in the distribution of treatment outcomes increases patients' value, a phenomenon we call "the value of hope."
- The willingness of people to trade life expectancy for HRQoL improvement (or vice versa) varies with the baseline HRQoL.

For these reasons, we believe that widespread implementation of the GRACE method to value medical interventions would improve the well-being of populations throughout the world. It would better align centralized or decentralized decisions about treatment value with the actual values held by people in those populations. This book is designed to help people better understand the GRACE method and how to implement it.

The GRACE approach is still new, and (at this writing) no actual evaluations of medical interventions have been published using the GRACE approach. The reason is simple: We do not yet have published estimates of some key data, particularly how much people have diminishing returns to health and how risk averse, or even risk-preferring, they are regarding uncertain health outcomes. One goal of this book is to stimulate the creation of the new knowledge necessary to fully implement our approach.

We hope both that you enjoy reading our book and that it helps you begin to use GRACE in your professional capacity, whether as a student studying CEA, an academic or consultant conducting research to measure value of new and existing medical interventions, or a professional working within a biopharmaceutical company or medical device company helping guide investments in alternative research areas or to establish value for products entering the market.

Various sections of this book have precise mathematical formulations with a series of specific definitions of terms. Some of these measure statistical properties of outcomes of medical interventions. Others measure people's preferences regarding specifically how HRQoL creates economists' "utility." Following this Preface, you will find a compendium of the terms we use throughout this book, conveniently located (we intend) for easy and rapid access as you read through the book.

ACKNOWLEDGMENTS

We acknowledge the continuously effective and valuable research support from Hanh Nguyen, our colleague at the University of Southern California's Leonard D. Schaeffer Center for Health Policy and Economics. We also acknowledge the careful review of the mathematical derivations and calculations throughout the book by Drishti Baid, Lukas Hager, Devin Incerti, and Karen Mulligan.

GENERAL ACRONYMS AND ABBREVIATIONS

GRACE: The generalized risk-adjusted cost-effectiveness model for valuing health improvement.

HTA: Health technology assessment

C: The value of consumption, defined as income (Y) minus medical expenses.

T: "Treatment" therapy, the new treatment being evaluated. Often appears as a subscript.

C: In a different context, "comparison" or "control" therapy to which T is compared. Often appears as a subscript.

H: "Health," the summary measure of well-being in the dimension of HRQoL.

$V(C, H)$: The value (utility) a person derives for various levels of consumption (C) and health (H). In our work, we specifically separate this so that $V(C, H) = U(C)W(H)$, where $U(C)$ is the utility derived from consumption and $W(H)$ is the well-being (utility) derived from H.

CEA: Cost-effectiveness analysis, as defined in Garber and Phelps (1997).

QALY: Quality-adjusted life year, A summary measure of overall gains in LE and HRQoL as used in standard CEA.

WTP: Willingness to pay for health care improvements.

HRQoL: Health-related quality of life, typically measured on a 0–1 scale.

LE: Life expectancy.

CRRA: Constant relative risk aversion, wherein risk aversion does not vary with H or C.

IRRA: Increasing relative risk aversion, wherein risk aversion increases with H or C.

DRRA: Decreasing relative risk aversion, wherein risk aversion declines with increases in H or C.

HARA: Hyperbolic absolute risk aversion model (CRRA is a special case).

MRS: The marginal rate or substitution between any two goods. In GRACE, this typically refers to the MRS between HRQoL and LE.

UTILITY (PREFERENCE) PARAMETERS REGARDING QUALITY OF LIFE

ω_C (omega-C): The elasticity of utility with respect to consumption (C).

ω_H (omega-H): The elasticity of utility with respect to health (H).

K: WTP per QALY in standard CEA, defined as $K = \dfrac{C}{\omega_C}$.

K_{GRACE}: WTP per QALY using the GRACE method with no disability.

K_{GRACE}^{D}: K_{GRACE} when incorporating non-zero baseline disability.

r_H^* (r-star-H): The relative risk aversion in health, defined as

$$r_H^* = -\frac{HW''(H)}{W'(H)},$$

where $W'(H)$ is the first derivative of $W(H)$ and $W''(Hs)$ is the second derivative of $W(H)$.

π_H^* (pi-star-H): Relative prudence in H, defined as

$$\pi_H^* = -\frac{HW'''(H)}{W''(H)},$$

where $W'''(H)$ is the third derivative of $W(H)$.

τ_H^* (tau-star-H): Relative temperance in H, defined as

$$\tau_H^* = -\frac{HW''''(H)}{W'''(H)},$$

where $W''''(H)$ is the fourth derivative of $W(H)$.

STATISTICAL PARAMETERS

ϕ (phi): The probability of an acute illness occurring in period 1.

p_1 (p-one): The probability of survival from period 0 to period 1.

σ_T^2 (sigma-squared-T): Variance of health outcomes, as measured in HRQoL in the T group.

σ_C^2 (sigma-squared-C): Variance of health outcomes, as measured in HRQoL in the C group.

γ_1 (gamma-1): Pearson's coefficient of skewness (can be subscripted as T or C).

γ_2 (gamma-2): Pearson's coefficient of kurtosis (can be subscripted as T or C).

$\Delta\sigma^2$: The difference in variance between treatment (T) and comparison (C) therapies.

HEALTH AND TREATMENT VALUES

B: Stochastic HRQoL gain ("benefit").

μ_B: The average gain in HRQoL from using T relative to C. $\mu_B = E(B)$.

μ_P: Average increase in probability of survival from T relative to C.

μ_H: Mean HRQoL level in the sick state if untreated.

H_0: Baseline level of HRQoL, often assumed to equal to 1.0.

H_{1S}: Stochastic level of HRQoL in period 1 if sick; μ_H is the expected value of H_{1S}.

H_{1W}: Stochastic non-sick HRQoL level in period 1, including any permanent disability.

ℓ^* (l-star): The relative loss in HRQoL due to untreated disease (measured on a 0 to 1 scale).

d^* (d-star): The relative loss in HRQoL due to permanent disability (measured on a 0 to 1 scale).

t^* (t-star): The relative loss in HRQoL from treated acute illness measured on a 0 to 1 scale).

H_{0d}: Actual level of HRQoL in period 0 if disabled; $H_{0d} = H_0(1 - d^*)$.

μ_T: Average treated HRQoL outcome; $\mu_T = \mu_H + \mu_B$.

CALCULATED PARAMETERS IN GRACE

R: The disease-severity multiplier, defined as the ratio (hence "R") of the marginal utility of HRQoL in the untreated sick state to the marginal utility of HRQoL in the well state.

ε (epsilon): The number of deterministic HRQoL units that equal the value of each unit gain in average HRQoL. When risk aversion equals 0, $\varepsilon = 1$.

δ (delta): The MRS between LE and HRQoL.

ρ (rho): A parameter used to calculate δ. See Chapter 4.

ψ (psi): The Taylor series summary measure that captures diminishing returns to HRQoL in the context of valuing the effect of disability on utility.

$D = \dfrac{1}{1 - \psi d^*}$: The summary measure of the effect of disability on WTP.

Why We Need Cost-Effectiveness Analysis, How It Is Done, and Why It Needs Fixing

What God has joined together, let no one separate.

—MARK 10:9

WHY DO WE NEED COST-EFFECTIVENESS ANALYSIS?

The Wedge Between Value and Cost

It may seem odd to start a discussion of cost-effectiveness analysis (CEA) with this question, but the proper approach begins with an understanding of the unique "marketplace" for medical care—treatments by doctors, nurses, therapists of various specialization, and dentists; hospital care; emergency room visits; urgent care; prescription drugs; medical devices; and others. Unlike any other good or service that one can imagine, the link between "value" and "cost to the consumer" has been shattered when we think about medical care.

The source of this disconnection, of course, is health insurance, whether provided through national health plans (as in the United Kingdom and elsewhere); government-provided insurance (as in Canada); or provided

Valuing Health. Charles E. Phelps and Darius N. Lakdawalla, Oxford University Press. © Oxford University Press 2024.
DOI: 10.1093/oso/9780197686287.003.0001

through regulated private insurance markets of various types, such as in the United States and many European and other nations. The methods of financing the health insurance do not matter significantly for the problem at hand. Stated simply, health insurance, no matter how financed, disconnects the prices people pay at the time of use for medical care from the cost of producing it. The link between price and value is gone.

In standard economic markets, whether competitive or monopolized or anything in between, costs of production affect the prices charged, and consumers choose to purchase the items sold in such markets if they receive at least as much value from the purchase as the "going rate" price. But with health insurance, the price consumers see is often much lower than the cost of production and sometimes even near or at zero. This divergence between price and cost affects patients' choices regarding when to seek or use medical care and, if using care, how much (Newhouse et al., 1996), with fully insured patients using as much as 50% more than those without insurance.

There is good reason for buying health insurance: The variability of illness and injury creates large financial risks for people, and obtaining health insurance to protect against such risks is a logical and desirable outcome. Recent analyses show that, by far, the dominant factor in choosing health insurance coverage is the magnitude of the financial risk created by highly variable illness and injury risk (Phelps, 2022a).

Most other types of insurance reimburse people for losses they have suffered with cash payments that can be used for any purpose. If your home burns down, the insurer pays you an estimate of its value, but you do not have to rebuild the home to its exact former specifications to receive the insurance payment. You can move into a smaller home and pay for your children's education, or you can even buy a seagoing catamaran and live aboard it, traveling around the world.

Similarly, if you get into a fender-bender, you can use the insurance payment to fix the vehicle, or you can drive around a ROHOTM[1] and build up your wine cellar collection. The existence of markets offering this type of insurance rests on the ability of insurers to assess the value of the object (and damage thereto) using reliable market measures such as the cost of similar homes or cars or using estimates from general contractors (for homes) or mechanics (for vehicles) of the cost of repair. However— and this is a key distinction—the insurance company pays for the damage or loss in a fixed amount, and you are free to use the proceeds in any way you wish.

Health insurance works quite differently. There is no effective mechanism for insurers to assess the value of a health loss. How much does a year's living with Alzheimer disease or unrelenting sciatic nerve pain or migraine headaches or acute depression "cost" a particular individual? The insurer would struggle to determine this for its beneficiaries.[2] Therefore, health insurance uses a different method to reduce the financial risk associated with random illnesses and injuries. It pays for the medical care used to relieve the problem, thereby reducing the price, sometimes to zero, sometimes to a copayment per "visit" or "hospitalization." The overall effect is unambiguous, and it occurs no matter whether the health insurance comes from a central national plan, a market-based system, or mix-and-match systems that predominate throughout the world. The link between value and cost to the consumer has been severed.

Consequences: Some Medical Care Has Minimal Value

This severing of value and cost leads to what others have called "flat-of-the-curve" medicine because it may sometimes produce minimal marginal value. Medical care can have enormous benefit in improving HRQoL and extending LE. But the *average* value tells us nothing about the incremental value of extending those valuable services to increasingly wider sets of patients with increasingly equivocal symptoms that the treatment might improve. That requires an understanding of the "marginal value" of expanding the use of the treatment.

This expansion of use can occur along two dimensions that economists call the "extensive" and "intensive" margins (Phelps, 1997). Consider as examples breast cancer screening for women (mammography) or prostate cancer screening (tests measuring prostate-specific antigen [PSA]) for men. Medical practitioners must make two decisions about offering such tests: the ages of eligibility (the extensive margin) and frequency of the test (the intensive margin).[3] For example, the U.S. Preventive Services Task Force (USPSTF), the body charged with recommending use of preventive services in the United States, recommends PSA testing for men aged 55–69 years and against testing for men aged 70 years or older. The USPSTF recommends biennial mammography screening for women aged 50–74 years. Changing the frequency from "biennial" to some other rate, e.g., "yearly," would be a change on the intensive margin.

In contrast, the prestigious Mayo Clinic recommends annual screening (the extensive margin) for women beginning at age 40 years, not age 50 years as the USPSTF recommends. Similarly, the American Cancer Society recommends annual screening starting at age 40 years and considers biennial screening appropriate for women older than age 55 years.

An early and highly influential study in the prestigious *British Medical Journal* (Williams, 1985) highlighted this issue in the specific use of coronary bypass surgeries. Williams' Table III, abstracted here in Table 1.1, demonstrates this issue vividly. This reveals two important issues. First, reading from top to bottom, the more severe the disease, the lower the cost per quality-adjusted life year (QALY) gained (the right-hand column) for coronary artery bypass grafting (CABG). In every category of disease severity (how clogged the arteries were), single-vessel disease was vastly more expensive per QALY than more complicated (double or triple) disease, and disease in the left main artery offered the greatest "bang for the buck" from CABG.

The other issue is that choice of technology mattered. For single-vessel disease, the opportunity existed for using a new technology (percutaneous transluminal coronary angioplasty [PTCA]) instead of CABG. For single-vessel disease at every level of severity, PTCA reduced the cost per QALY by about a factor of four compared with traditional open-heart surgery.

Most medical procedures are subject to the same kinds of uncertainty about value. But it is an iron-clad fact that as use of any intervention

Table 1.1 Williams' Estimates of Cost per QALY for
Coronary Artery Interventions

Degree of Angina	Anatomic Area	Treatment	ICER (£1,000)
Severe	Left main	CABG	1.04
	Triple vessel	CABG	1.27
	Double vessel	CABG	2.28
	One vessel	CABG	11.4
	One vessel	PTCA	2.4
Moderate	Left main	CABG	1.33
	Triple vessel	CABG	2.4
	Double vessel	CABG	4
	One vessel	CABG	12
	One vessel	PTCA	3.4
Mild	Left main	CABG	2.52
	Triple vessel	CABG	6.3
	Double vessel	CABG	12.6
	One vessel	CABG	—
	One vessel	PTCA	10.72

CABG, coronary artery bypass grafting; ICER, incremental cost-effectiveness ratio;
PTCA, percutaneous transluminal coronary angioplasty.

source: Data from Williams (1985).

expands, either on the intensive or the extensive margin, the expected incremental benefit necessarily falls.

Figure 1.1 shows this phenomenon, graphing total benefit versus total number of treatments for any "typical" medical intervention's use at the population level. The idea is that technologies are first used in cases in which they can produce the greatest benefit. But as their use expands (on the intensive or extensive margin or both), the marginal new patient treated derives increasingly less benefit. Graphically, the *marginal* benefit rate is the slope of the curve in Figure 1.1 shown in the long-dashed line, whereas the *average* benefit (at the same level of use) is the slope of the short-dashed line. At low levels of use, the marginal benefit can be quite

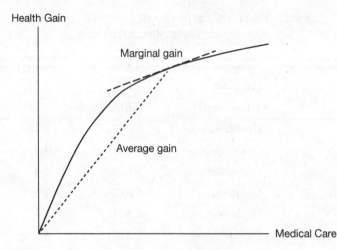

Figure 1.1 Typical health gains as medical care use expands on the extensive or intensive margins.

high. At high levels of use, the marginal benefit (the slope of the curve) can become almost flat, indicating little or no incremental gain in health benefit as the number of treatments expands.

At low levels of use, the marginal benefit (the slope of the tangent line) exceeds the average benefit. Conversely, at high levels of use, as shown in Figure 1.1, the marginal benefit is lower than the average benefit—the slope is flatter. This is an important distinction. Saying that a treatment has "minimal incremental benefit" does not mean that it is useless on average. The average benefit can be large. But when deciding about the proper use of the intervention on the extensive and intensive margins, the average benefit is not useful for decision-making. Only the incremental (marginal) benefit matters. In other words, when deciding whether or not to treat another patient, what matters is the potential benefit to that patient, not to the average for all patients who were previously treated. Proper CEA methods focus on incremental (marginal) benefits of treatments, not their average.

"Flat-of-the-curve medicine" describes the situation at the upper right corner of Figure 1.1. Adding more and more treatment, whether through expansion on the intensive or extensive margins, increasingly yields less and less incremental benefit. In a recent summary of technological innovation in medical care, a pair of leading health economists in the United States said that insured patients have "commonly received any medical advance that promised more than a *de minimis* benefit" (Chernew and Newhouse, 2012, p. 37). This almost necessarily occurs when insured patients pay little or nothing for their care, and mostly they do not even remotely know the cost of services provided to them.

We can make use of this concept by measuring the incremental costs required to achieve an incremental benefit of improved health. This is known as the incremental cost-effectiveness ratio (ICER). It measures added costs in the local currency (dollars, Euros, British pound sterling, pesos, rials, yuan, rupees, yen, etc.) and typically measures benefits in a combined metric known as QALYs.[4] QALYs combine improvements of HRQoL and additions to LE. Subsequent chapters analyze the composition of a QALY and the value of benefits of HRQoL and LE improvements using important new methods to understand "value." For now, we need only to think about QALYs as a composite good, just as "food" is a composite good consisting of many specific types of food and dining experiences, and "transportation" encompasses planes, trains, automobiles, bicycles, subway systems, and many other ways to travel.

A Proxy for Market Valuation

We now come to the crux of this chapter: Because health insurance has severed the link between consumers' appreciation of value and the prices that they pay to acquire any given treatment, many situations arise in which it would be desirable to construct a proxy to assess what incremental value arises from expanding the use of an existing treatment or replacing existing treatments, diagnostic tests, or preventive interventions. The current "standard" for doing this throughout the world is the ICER—the ratio of incremental cost to incremental gains in health.

In best practice, CEAs carefully measure the health benefits of the new technology (typically measured in QALYs in some specific way) compared with the next-best alternative (the "comparator" or "control" therapy).

Similarly, they compare the costs of treating patients using the new treatment (T) versus the comparison or control (C).

The control might be the current standard of care for any specific intervention or (if no treatments exist) the consequences of "doing nothing." These need not be costless. For example, patients with progressive neurological diseases will incur increasing medical costs for ongoing care and life support, even if no "treatment" exists that might alter the course of their disease.

The ICER provides a widely used basis for decision-making about using the intervention. Doing so requires that the decision-making body adopt a specific threshold of the maximum willingness to pay (WTP) to gain 1 QALY. The acceptable cost per QALY determines which innovations achieve coverage in health insurance plans or are included in the service package.

Knowing the ICER for any use of a medical intervention can guide many important decisions, both private and public. For private health insurance plans, applying CEA methods can help guide coverage decisions in their offerings to the general public.

One obvious use of CEA exists in a set of organizations (both private and public) that directly treat patients for their illnesses instead of paying for treatment provided by independent providers. In the United States, these are called health maintenance organizations (HMOs), the Kaiser-Permanente network of health plans being a well-known example. The U.S. government operates a series of similar plans for select populations, including the Indian Health Service; the U.S. Department of Veterans Affairs' hospital system; and (combined with related health insurance plans) the military health care systems of the U.S. Army, Navy, and Air Force.

Probably the best-known example of a national health plan is the National Health Service (NHS) of the United Kingdom. More precisely, four separate plans exist: the NHS in England, NHS Scotland, NHS Wales, and Health and Social Care in Northern Ireland. NHS and NHS Wales operate with general guidance from the National Institute for Health and Care Excellence (NICE) as to which medical treatments will be offered to enrollees. NICE, more than any other organization in the world, formally uses CEA to determine which medical interventions will be included in the NHS "package."

NICE serves in the United Kingdom as a proxy to estimate value to consumers of various medical interventions and then compares the ICER to a "threshold value" to determine whether or not to include interventions in the package of covered services. NICE formally operates with a threshold of £20,000–£30,000 per QALY, where the current per capita gross domestic product (GDP) is approximately £30,000. Separately, the UK Department of the Treasury recommends using thresholds of £60,000 per QALY for assessing environmental projects that improve health— approximately 2× per capita GDP.

In the United States, a private organization, the Institute for Clinical and Economic Review (ICER), evaluates new medical interventions and uses a range of thresholds of $50,000 to $200,000 per QALY; the per capita GDP was approximately $65,000 in 2020, so their threshold range is a slightly expanded range of 1× to 3× per capita GDP. This closely matches previous recommendations from the World Health Organization (WHO) and also the American College of Cardiology and American Heart Association, which support the 1× to 3× per capita GDP recommendation from WHO.[5]

What Matters Here

It must be remember that what is really at stake here is people's willingness to pay for improving their health, at the cost of foregone consumption of other goods and services. A number of approaches exist to determining the optimal WTP; some of them very ad hoc, and some are fully grounded in economic theory.[6] They seem to converge (to pick a specific interval for discussion) at about 2× or 3× per capita GDP as a single "national" rule (as for the British NHS). However, there remains considerable disagreement about the best methods to make this determination and hence the "correct" threshold value.

To complicate things even further, some people argue that it is not foregone consumption of other goods and services that matters but, rather, foregone use of other health care interventions. This situation arises when the health care system (e.g., the British NHS) operates with a predetermined fixed budget, perhaps inefficiently determined from a broader societal perspective, but nevertheless a binding budget constraint. In that setting, decision-making occurs within the budget constraint, and in that world, foregone benefits of other medical interventions determine the proper decision threshold.

Nevertheless, there is widespread agreement that where K is the predetermined cutoff (threshold) for acceptable ICERs, the proper use of CEA is to employ or reimburse, depending on the setting, any medical intervention for which

$$\frac{\text{Incremental Cost}}{\text{Incremental Health Gain}} \leq K \qquad (1.1)$$

Specifically, the ideal protocol, where possible, is to increase on the extensive or intensive margin or both until Eq. (1.1) is an exact equality.

The general point to be made here is that CEA provides a proxy measure of value when market-based measures are unreliable. That unreliability arises when extensive insurance coverage shatters the link between value and price to consumers of the relevant product. Health care provides the quintessential example of such a situation. The related concept of benefit–cost analysis has widespread use in various areas, most importantly in the arena of environmental projects and other "public goods" where market failure exists.

We also note that CEA and our more general model, the generalized and risk-adjusted cost-effectiveness (GRACE) model, have potential application in multiple areas of decision-making. The basic formulation assesses the value from the standpoint of adding access to a technology in a health care system, particularly people's WTP for such access. Decisions such as this can be made in system-wide health plans such as the British NHS or when determining whether to cover a medical intervention in a private or public health insurance plan in situations with market-based insurance coverage. These types of decisions regularly must be made with respect to prescription drugs in the creation of "formulary" lists of approved drugs or when determining the pricing "tier" at which a drug will be placed.

CEA can also be used to help patients think through the choice among competing treatments for diseases that have befallen them. In the more general conception of CEA (e.g., for use at health-plan levels), both the probability of survival and the probability of acquiring a specific disorder or disease enter the analysis. However, setting these probabilities to 1.0 (certainty about the disease event) puts the CEA model into the perspective of choosing among alternative treatments—for example, for a specific type of cancer. In these models, the appropriate "price" in the evaluation is the co-payment that patients must make, unless patients take on a wider societal view and include the actual costs of various treatments.

HOW TO PERFORM COST-EFFECTIVENESS ANALYSIS

In this section, we give a brief overview about how a typical CEA study is constructed. For a comprehensive review, see the second edition of *Cost-Effectiveness in Health and Medicine* by Neumann et al. (2017).

When evaluating a new technology, the first step is to choose the proper comparator ("control") therapy, which we dub "C." Everything we measure about the new therapy "T" will be compared with C. For some medical conditions, C will be the current standard of care, which may have a number of alternatives from which to choose. If data are available, C would desirably be the alternative with the most favorable ICER among the available alternatives. If some doubt exists, analyses of T can include several comparators in their studies. For some other medical conditions, no standard of care therapy will exist. In these cases, C is "doing nothing," but in most cases, "doing nothing" at a minimum can involve palliative care and considerable caretaker burden, which should be included as a cost of "doing nothing."

The ICER is a standard formula, comparing the added costs of using T (compared with C) and measures the added health gains, typically measured in QALYs. Then the ICER is

$$\text{ICER}_T = \frac{\left[\text{Cost}_T - \text{Cost}_C \right]}{\left[\text{QALY}_T - \text{QALY}_C \right]} = \frac{\Delta \text{Cost}}{\Delta \text{QALY}} \qquad (1.2)$$

This is the same concept as in Eq. (1.1) with a bit more detail added.

The data needed to measure "cost" accurately typically involve creating a catalog of all medical interventions used by the T and C patients, not only as part of the therapy but also in subsequent treatments that, for example, might involve adverse events associated with T or C. With the assembled list of medical interventions that patients receive in each arm of the study, the measure of "cost" then emerges by applying a "price" to each unit of treatment received. Therein lies a problem (and one that we shall not solve herein): Measuring "price" is fraught with difficulties.

In pure HMO plans such as Kaiser-Permanente, there is no direct need to attach prices to the services provided to enrollees. However, the medical record systems of such organizations commonly have quite comprehensive evidence on all medical care usage because the systems are "closed" and patients receive all of their care within the same system. Hence, all events are recorded in the same medical record. In concept, such organizations can also calculate the incremental cost of providing each medical intervention, using, for example, standard concepts from industrial engineering. From these data, they could estimate the ICER for any intervention.

With regard to fee-for-service systems, common in the United States and elsewhere, the concept of "price" remains fuzzy. U.S. hospitals, for example, commonly have a set of prices on file, but almost nobody ever pays them. A common "bill" for a simple surgical procedure might include $40,000 in "billed charges," $5,500 in "approved charges" by the health insurance plan involved, and perhaps $500 in co-payment due from the patient. The $40,000 number is a fiction, used by hospitals to "price out" their charity care (some amount of which they must provide to maintain their not-for-profit status).[7]

In this sort of transaction, where does the $5,500 in approved charges come from? Each separate health insurance plan in the United States has a set of charges the insurer agrees to pay, and in most cases, that insurer has contracts with numerous hospitals that specify the approved charges for every activity the hospital undertakes. Unfortunately, these price lists are not generally available to the public and hence cannot generally be used as a proxy for costs.

Since January 2021, U.S. law requires all hospitals to disclose their prices, with detail (as specified on the Center for Medicare and Medicaid Services' website) to include "gross charges, discounted cash prices, payer-specific negotiated charges, and de-identified minimum and maximum negotiated charges." The "gross charges" are the quasi-fictious "list prices" discussed in the previous paragraph. "Discounted cash prices" represent the average price for non-insured patients after the hospital provides a discount of some sort, often negotiated on a case-by-case basis. Here, "payer-specific negotiated charges" are the approved charges described in the previous paragraph and constitute the large bulk of services provided to patients who do not have Medicare or Medicaid coverage.

The negotiated prices are highly protected. A 2021 study found that only approximately half of all U.S. hospitals posted their "cash prices" and only 1 in 20 provided the legally required "minimum negotiated prices."[8] This was not simple neglect to fulfill their obligations to the law but, rather, a deliberate process to hide their price data.[9]

Although many approaches exist, given the "invisibility" of private-insurance transactions prices, most health care researchers in the United States fall back on approved payments by the U.S. Medicare program as a proxy for "cost." Although Medicare is often thought of as a plan for those older than age 65 years, its coverage of people with permanent disabilities requires it to have payment schedules for virtually every medical procedure available, including, to the surprise of many people, pediatric and obstetric procedures.

Many other approaches are available, and vast literatures exist discussing the "best" way to measure costs of health care. We do not attempt to enumerate these here, let alone describe how to undertake these alternatives. For further detail on this issue, see Chapter 8 of Neumann et al. (2017).

Measuring the QALY side of the ledger is very familiar to people conducting health economics and outcomes research. The "gold standard" is a randomized controlled trial (RCT), wherein patients are randomly assigned to receive either T or C, and then all patients are followed for a sufficient length of time, depending on the disease and treatment, to accumulate evidence on their health status and, as pertinent, death. These studies select various possible health outcomes and then, in the course of the study, measure the probabilities that each possible outcome occurs. The "expected health outcome" can then be calculated from these data.

When RCT data are not available, numerous studies now use prospective or retrospective panel data or a growing body of approaches generally known as "real-world data." The benefits and risks of these approaches constitute an entire new range of analysis within the broader field of health technology assessment (HTA).

The basic concept for comparing the possible outcomes associated with two treatments can be captured in a decision tree. The tree visually portrays the possible outcome pathways that follow a treatment choice, the probabilities at each junction point along the pathways, and the costs and health outcomes at the end of each possible pathway of outcomes. The goal of an RCT or comparable analysis is to measure all of the relevant probabilities and the outcomes at the end of each branch of the decision tree. A very simple decision tree might look something like that shown in Figure 1.2.

In this simple example, the solid "box" is a decision point, where the upper arm is a decision to treat (e.g., to undergo surgery) and the lower arm is to "do nothing." At the end of each branch of the tree, the costs and health outcomes (C and H, respectively) of each pathway are shown. Each node (represented by a circle) represents a probabilistic event. In many cases, more than two possible outcomes exist at some of the nodes. These data form the basis for the "incremental" costs and health outcomes analysis because the decision tree allows us to compute the differences in expected costs and expected health outcomes between the two choices under consideration. In this case, the comparison would be the potential outcomes and costs of the single treatment versus the (known) costs and outcomes of "no treat."

As a baseline outcome, assume that "no treat" leaves the patient with a HRQoL of 0.6. and an annual cost of $5,000 per year (e.g., costs of home health aides to assist in living). This means that a complete cure creates 0.4 gain in HRQoL per year of remaining lifetime in health outcomes.

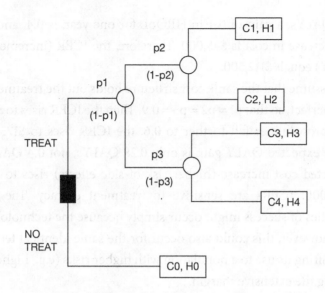

Figure 1.2 An example of a highly simplified decision tree allowing calculation of ICER values for different combinations of parameters.

Initially, assume that if the treatment works fully (with probability $p1 = 1$) and has no side effects (with probability $p2 = p3 = 1$), it returns the patient to full health, so $H1 = 1$ on a $[0,1]$ interval to measure HRQoL. However, if the treatment also has the risk of side effects (with $p2 < 1$) that permanently reduce HRQoL by 0.1, then the expected health outcome and costs change.

If the treatment is fully successful but the side effect occurs, the final health outcome is $H2 = 1 - 0.1 = 0.9$ HRQoL. Assume also that this incurs an additional cost to deal with the side effect, C5, so $C2 = C1 + C5$. This makes the treatment less favorable because net health gains fall and costs rise.

In our example decision tree, there is also the possibility [with probability of $(1 - p1)$] that the treatment might work with only 50% efficacy. In this case, the health gain is half of a "full cure," or a HRQoL gain of 0.2. Therefore, $H3 = 0.8$. Finally, the same side effect might occur even when the treatment only works with half of full efficacy, so $H4 = 0.7$. If this occurs, the same added costs occur to deal with the side effects, so $C4 = C3 + C5$.

This small "toy" decision tree illustrates the basic concepts in this chapter. Begin with simple assumptions that $C1 = C3 = \$50,000$ and $C5 = \$10,000$, so $C2 = C4 = \$60,000$. The simplest of all possible "decision trees" occurs when $p1 = p2 = 1$. In this case, the treatment is always perfect, the expected gain in QALYs, a gain of 0.4 in HRQoL for one year, is 0.4, and the expected increase in cost is $45,000. Therefore, the ICER (incremental cost per QALY) equals $112,500.

Now assume that the same cost structure holds but the treatment is not quite so perfect, so that $p1 = p2 = p3 = 0.9$. Then the ICER rises to $124,324. If those probabilities fall further to 0.6, the ICER rises to $175,000 because the expected QALY gain is only 0.28 QALYs, not 0.4 QALYs, and the expected cost increase (higher risk of side effects) rises to $49,000, not $45,000. ICERs are sensitive to treatment efficacy. The reduced probabilities of success might occur simply because the technology is not perfect; however, this could also occur for the same identical technology but by shifting its use to a population with higher risks (e.g., higher age), a shift along the extensive margin.

Now return to the base case of a perfect treatment, where $p1 = p2 = 1$. But now, raise the basic cost of the procedure to $75,000, not $50,000. In this case, the ICER is $175,000 (i.e., $70,000 added costs divided by 0.4 QALYs gained). With those same higher costs but the success probabilities of $p1 = p2 = p3 = 0.9$, the ICER rises still further to $191,892 per QALY.

Real-life decision trees are almost always far more complicated than this simple toy, but it reveals the basic concepts of the decision analysis models that underlie CEA. ICERs rise as expected treatment efficacy falls, and ICERs also rise (obviously) as treatment costs rise. More complex Markov multiperiod models require data measuring probabilities of transitioning from one state to another, period by period, for as long as the subjects are followed, but the basic concepts remain unchanged. These more complex models are now quite commonplace, as computing and relevant software provide advanced capabilities for carrying out such analyses, and advanced data collection techniques support the measurement of relevant transition probabilities in the Markov matrix.

Constructing decision trees typically requires specific medical knowledge about the relevant disease condition, available treatments and ways to measure their treatment efficacy, and a parallel capability to measure side effects and their consequences. Measurement of costs could well involve economists or other specialists in health services research with appropriate training. The statistical analyses (including calculating sample size to obtain desired power of testing) typically falls into the domain of statisticians, most commonly those specializing in studies such as these—biostatisticians. Underlying prior probabilities of disease and their outcomes may well require the input of clinical or population epidemiologists.

Carrying out good CEA studies requires teamwork, often with a wide array of scientific and clinical skills. This is not solo figure skating, in which each of the performers displays their specialized skills. It is ice hockey, a highly complex "team sport." It is not an unaccompanied singing solo; it is a highly complex orchestral/choral production.

As we shall show in later chapters, the skills, resources, and data collection necessary to carry out a full GRACE analysis do not differ importantly from those needed to conduct a standard CEA. Most of the "missing" elements needed by GRACE can be assembled from information already in the hands of analysts doing standard CEA studies. The only information that is truly "new" is measurement of the value parameters measuring how value to consumers changes with their levels of health and the extent of risk aversion to uncertain treatment outcomes. We discuss these issues in more detail in later chapters.

LIMITATIONS OF COST-EFFECTIVENESS ANALYSIS

Cost-effectiveness analysis has many built-in limitations, some of which GRACE shares and some of which it overcomes. Some of these limitations stem from the underlying methodology: Both standard CEA and GRACE rely on the values of a "representative individual" who seeks to maximize expected utility. This is a standard paradigm in economic analysis in general and the subfield of "welfare economics" into which cost–benefit and cost-effectiveness analysis fit. These models are limited by the set of "things" that are put into the representative individuals' utility function that might create value. The most basic of these functions states that "income" creates utility, in which case the utility function is $U = U(\text{Income})$. The field of labor economics was built in part by inserting "leisure" into the utility function, so that $U = U$(Income, Leisure). This allowed the study of people's labor supply decisions in new and insightful ways.

The field of health economics generally uses utility functions that include "consumption" of market goods and services and "health," which in turn is improved (perhaps imperfectly) by the use of various types of medical interventions. "Consumption" is defined as income minus medical spending. Therefore, the direct utility function is $U = U$(Consumption, Health), which leads into a more market-oriented "derived" utility function of $U = U$(Consumption, Medical Care). In this model, people do not buy medical care because it is intrinsically enjoyable but, rather, because it can improve health. Although the basic model leads to a "demand for health," as originally formulated by pioneer health economist Michael Grossman, this also leads to study of the "derived demand for medical care" (Grossman, 1972a, 1972b, 2000).

This leads us to the inherent deficiencies in both CEA and GRACE. If consumers value the health and economic well-being of others in addition to their own (i.e., they exhibit altruism), then there is no way to use CEA or GRACE to analyze these preferences for altruism. The same is true of "scientific spillovers" that have value to future generations or others alive today. Economic models based on individuals' utility cannot generally deal with "externalities" in economics—situations in which a consumer's decision influences the well-being of others, whose welfare they do not consider when determining their own "best actions."

Within the domain of health economics, other areas involving externalities include vaccination status, face mask wearing, and participation in clinical studies that help inform others about the value of various medical interventions.[10] This health care domain also importantly includes the funding of "public health" agencies that oversee water safety and sewage disposal, epidemiologic studies and data provision, vaccination recommendations, and many other activities.

An ISPOR task force, of which we were both participants, laid out a now-famous (or infamous) "value flower," the "petals" of which showed various elements of value. Box 1.1 outlines these value elements, taken from one of the seven reports issued by this special task force (Lakdawalla et al., 2018).

Box 1.1

VALUE ELEMENTS FROM ISPOR

QALYS
Net cost
Adherence-improving factors
Productivity
Altruism[a]
Caregiver burden[a]
Fear of contagion
Value of knowing
Value of insurance
Severity of disease
Value of hope
Real option value
Equity
Scientific spillovers

[a]Not in the original ISPOR value flower.

Standard CEA incorporates only the first two of these in its basic structure. The second edition of *Cost-Effectiveness in Health and Medicine* (Neumann et al., 2017) offered precise ways to include "productivity," and the CEA structure readily allows analysts to incorporate adherence-improving factors and, by expanding the set of people affected by a disease, caregiver value. Issues of contagion can similarly be incorporated by expanding the list of "those affected" to all members of a society. But that set of value elements essentially is the limit of the range of traditional CEA.

By introducing diminishing returns into the model, GRACE provides ways to coherently incorporate the value of insurance, the value of hope, disease severity, and (although we have not done it formally) the value of knowing.[11] GRACE does this in a unified way, ensuring that there is no "double-counting" of these additional measures of value.

"Real option value" requires a separate type of information—the estimated probability that a treatment will keep a patient alive until a "cure" is found, which requires two distinct estimates: the probability that a new cure emerges within time T and the probability that the treatment will keep the patient alive to time T. A few estimates of this value appear in the literature, generally based on standard CEA models once the "probability of a cure being invented" is incorporated into the model (Snider et al., 2012; Sanchez et al., 2012; Li et al., 2019). Using GRACE-like measures to understand the differential value of curing severe illnesses would improve these models, but there is nothing particularly difficult about envisioning how to do this.

The next petal on the value flower is "equity." Despite the inherent limitations from using the utility function of a utility-maximizing individual, GRACE does offer some new insights into issues of equity, which we explore in Chapter 12.

This leaves the two value elements of "altruism" and "scientific spillovers." As noted above, neither standard CEA nor GRACE has an effective way of dealing with these issues. In some sense, they require separate measures of people's WTP for these values.

Particularly in the field of environmental economics, economists have devised a number of methods to elicit people's WTP for various improved environmental outcomes. The same is true for things generally considered as "public goods," wherein market equilibriums do not lead to efficient levels of production. National defense, public safety, and the production of information are obvious examples. In concept, the same could be done within the field of health care for the key issues of equity, in its many dimensions, and scientific spillovers. However, we believe that GRACE has nothing that uniquely illuminates these issues, and we therefore leave the analysis of these issues to others.

SUMMARY OF BOOK STRUCTURE

The remainder of this book discusses our new approach to valuation of medical interventions, the GRACE model. GRACE introduces declining returns to health into the value model. In so doing, it corrects the five errors of omission discussed in the Preface.

Chapter 2 of this book introduces the key concept of diminishing returns to health and the consequences of this simple but important change. Chapter 3 expands the analysis to include effects of uncertain treatment outcomes, which is important because of risk aversion in health, a consequence of diminishing returns in health. Chapter 4 then explores methods to combine changes in HRQoL and LE into a single comprehensive measure of value. Chapter 5 further extends that analysis to consider the effects of permanent disability on value of improving health.

The discussion in Chapters 2–5 rests on a simple two-period model—the "base period," in which decisions are made about future access to medical interventions, and "period 1," in which the individual may fall ill and which includes the value of any specific treatment provided in response to that illness. Chapter 6 extends GRACE from that simple two-period model, showing how to carry forward the implications of GRACE into multiperiod decision models with period-specific parameters and traditional discounting. This formulation extends GRACE, for example, to models using Monte Carlo simulations of multiperiod decision-making.

Neither CEA nor GRACE can be implemented in a decision context without decision-makers choosing a WTP threshold for comparison to cost-effectiveness estimates for individual technologies (in the traditional CEA approach) or generalizations of that concept that arise when introducing diminishing returns. Chapter 7 explores various ways to identify optimal decision thresholds and understand how they might vary across different settings.

The one "missing element" to conduct complete GRACE analyses is the estimation of the rate at which the returns to HRQoL gains diminish, or even increase, and the consequent implications for preferences over risky health outcomes. Chapter 8 assesses two different methods for estimating such preferences.

To bring all of the component parts together, Chapter 9 carries out a "worked example" of the model using hypothetical data. To do this completely requires estimates of people's attitude toward uncertainty in health outcomes and the rate at which the marginal utility of health gains changes. At this point in the development of GRACE, nobody has published estimates of these parameters. Furthermore, to our knowledge, nobody has published clinical data showing the variances and skewness in treatment outcomes of competing interventions that are needed to support a full GRACE analysis. Therefore, this analysis will necessarily use hypothetical data.

Chapter 10 assesses some transition issues for a health plan (or a society, more broadly) shifting from standard CEA-based methods to GRACE methodology. This chapter addresses currently used methods to adjust for illness severity, comparing their approaches to the GRACE methodology. Chapter 11 then explores the consequences of different combinations of the key GRACE parameters in a sensitivity analysis exercise, and it also discusses the potential implications on health plan "signals" sent to medical innovators about the value of health gains at different levels of illness severity.

Chapter 12 provides new insights on some implications of GRACE for ethical issues associated with evaluation of health technologies and the distribution of access to such technologies across various parts of the population. We discuss several potential avenues for considering ethical issues that GRACE might illuminate, and we compare two different approaches for valuing health care. The first is called welfarist economics (WE), of which GRACE is a family member. WE methods rely on individual utilities to measure value in the context of aggregate "social welfare functions." The alternative, called extra-welfarist economics, eschews use of individual valuations, preferring instead to substitute values derived from political or similar processes.

Chapter 13 concludes by summarizing the main issues raised by GRACE and the steps necessary to fully implement these concepts in formal HTA. These include a series of "done once" measurements of individual preferences about health care and risk aversion, and a series of data-reporting steps for organizations conducting specific technology evaluations, all of which should be readily accessible from data used to conduct current HTA studies.

Diminishing Returns . . . Everywhere

> External goods have a limit, like any other instrument, and all things useful are of such a nature that where there is too much of them, they must either do harm, or at any rate be of no use.
>
> —ARISTOTLE (*Politics*, Book 7, Chapter 1)

HEALTH OR THE UTILITY OF HEALTH?

We begin this chapter with a perhaps mundane but nevertheless important topic. We need to make clear what our generalized risk-adjusted cost-effectiveness (GRACE) model analysis focuses on, and how other approaches to these issues may cause some confusion. The question here is, What do we mean by quality-adjusted life year (QALY)?

According to the second edition of *Cost-Effectiveness in Health and Medicine* (Neumann et al., 2017), "Most CEA [cost-effectiveness analysis] analysts consider QALYs as measures of health" (p. 52). The UK's National Institute for Health and Care Excellence (NICE, 2022) uses the following definition: "[a] measure of the state of health of a person or group in which the benefits, in terms of length of life, are adjusted to reflect the quality of life." Note that there is no reference to the "utility" of health, just "the state of health." Neumann et al. (2017) further state that "for those who aspire

Valuing Health. Charles E. Phelps and Darius N. Lakdawalla, Oxford University Press. © Oxford University Press 2024.
DOI: 10.1093/oso/9780197686287.003.0002

to connect QALYs to utility theory, a number of important issues must be addressed" (p. 52). Indeed, these issues have created confusion in the practice of CEA.

Several CEA theorists have recognized that patients may have risk preferences over QALYs, even though these are not explicitly measured. These approaches rely on the standard result from expected utility theory that consumers remain risk-neutral in the level of utility, even if risk-averse over levels of consumption and health. To implement these "expected utility" models, analysts convert measures of health into measures of utility using "standard gamble" or other methods.[1] From this perspective, the incremental cost-effectiveness ratio must be interpreted as incremental costs per unit gain in health-related *utility*. In principle, this allows for risk aversion over HRQoL. In practice, "standard gamble" conversions have only modest test–retest reliability, and the outcomes differ significantly depending on whether chained gambles or basic reference gambles are used (Rutten-van Mouken et al., 1995; Law et al., 1998).

GRACE solves this problem by using measures of health, not utility, as inputs and then explicitly accounts for how declining marginal utility and risk aversion in health affect valuation. The key point here is that when we say "HRQoL," we mean a measure of health itself, without any attempt to convert the health index into a utility index. QALYs are typically defined as the product of the duration of a given health state, commonly life expectancy (LE) times the HRQoL. GRACE can rely on any measure of the HRQoL that meets our general criteria, namely the index from 0 to 1. Strictly speaking, GRACE does not employ standard QALYs, and it relaxes several of its rigid (and likely false) assumptions about preferences.

One way to acquire a direct measure of health is the traditional visual analog scale, wherein people mark a continuous line (or give a verbal number) measuring the intensity of pain that they are currently suffering. This does not ask for the utility associated with the pain but, rather, the level of pain itself. This is commonly used in clinical settings (with the meaning of the numbers reversed) wherein clinicians ask patients to rate their pain on a 0 to 10 scale, 10 being the worst ever felt, and 0 being "no pain." This measures the pain level directly, not the utility associated with it.

One example of the possible dimensions of "health" that might be used in an overall measure of health is the widely used EQ-5D measure from Europe.[2] It assesses health in five domains (mobility, self-care, usual activities, pain/suffering, and anxiety/depression), each rated on a 5-point severity scale (none, slight, moderate, severe, and extreme). Each of these is a measure of health, not its utility. They can be combined into a single scalar measure of health by assessing the relative importance of each domain—for example, using multi-criteria decision analysis models while still preserving the intent of our health status measure (Phelps and Madhavan, 2017). Judging from the frequency of direct-to-consumer advertisements on U.S. television, one might readily add several other dimensions of health to overall health measures, including sexual activity and physical appearance.

WHAT ARE DIMINISHING RETURNS AND WHY DO THEY MATTER?

Willingness to Pay for Health Gains as Measured by Foregone Consumption

With a clear understanding of the basic "input" to the GRACE model, we can now turn to perhaps the most central issue that GRACE illuminates: How does utility vary with the level of health? Economists have for many centuries thought about proper methods to measure "value." The standard tool for this is called the utility function.[3] It measures how happy people are and how income (or the goods and services one can buy with it) increase utility. Utility is difficult to directly measure because it cannot be seen, weighed, or measured.[4] Nevertheless, economists have figured out a number of ways to understand how utility is created and the observable consequences that flow from these ideas.

One of the most basic tools in this line of analysis—the marginal rate of substitution (MRS)—emerges as a very useful tool to think about how the "threshold" for CEA should be estimated. Let's begin with a simple example, in which "happiness" or "utility" is created by only two goods, perhaps the proverbial "apples and oranges," but it could also be bundles of other goods, such as "food" and "shelter" or "fine wines" and "winter skiing." To be neutral, we'll just call them $X1$ and $X2$. Then, we have the utility $U(X1, X2)$ that transforms people's consumption of $X1$ and $X2$ into a total measure of happiness (utility).

The MRS describes how budget-constrained people might make trade-offs between $X1$ and $X2$: Getting more $X2$ means giving up some $X1$. This involves analyzing different combinations of $X1$ and $X2$ that create the same level of happiness. Figure 2.1 portrays these trade-offs.

The curves in Figure 2.1 are bowed as shown because of the most fundamental axiom of economic analysis: People have diminishing returns to consuming any specific good or service. If you have two apples today, a third adds some value, but if you have 100 apples today, you would probably prefer trading some of them for a bottle of fine wine, a take-out

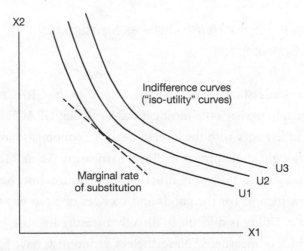

Figure 2.1 Typical graph of combinations of two economic "goods" that create the same level of utility (indifference curves). The slope of the curve at any point along it gives the marginal rate of substitution. Going outward from the origin, each curve shows a higher level of utility.

hamburger meal, or a ski lift ticket. People like variety, and they tend to avoid focusing their consumption on any single thing.

These curves are called iso-utility curves or, more commonly, indifference curves. All along each single curve, consumers do not care which combination of $X1$ and $X2$ they have because each creates the same level of happiness. People are "indifferent" across any two combinations of goods that lie on a single curve. In Figure 2.1, each of the higher up curves shows a higher level of utility (so U3 > U2 > U1).

You have seen this idea before if you have ever used a topographical map. Each of the lines on a "topo map" represents the same elevation, and once you get accustomed to using them, you can figure out rapidly what the mountain or valley portrayed on the map looks like. One might call these "iso-altitude" lines because each line shows the same altitude along the terrain. Perhaps we might call the indifference curves in Figure 2.1 iso-attitude lines if we were prone to such tomfoolery.

This same approach can extend to "goods" that are not bought and sold in the market. The quintessential nonmarket "good" that economists discuss is "leisure," and much of the field of labor economics addresses the "labor–leisure" trade-off using concepts essentially identical to Figure 2.1.

The math involved in the concept of MRS is fairly simple (but it does involve a bit of calculus). The key issue is the "marginal utility" that people get from adding a tiny bit of $X1$ from their current position and the commensurate loss in utility from giving up a smidgen of $X2$ to allow the purchase of the additional $X1$. Because economists universally assume that people have positive but diminishing marginal utility in consumption for all normal economic "goods," the partial derivatives show that $U'(X1) > 0$ and $U'(X2) > 0$, but each of these gets smaller (the slopes shrink) as $X1$ and $X2$ increase. Thus, the second derivatives $U''(X1)$ and $U''(X2)$ are both negative. Those two attributes of a utility function define "positive but diminishing marginal utility"—positive first derivatives and negative second derivatives of the utility function.

In health economics, the relevant "goods" are commonly defined as consumption (C), usually measured as income (Y) minus medical care expenses, and health (H), usually defined on a [0, 1] scale such that 1 = perfect health and 0 is the worst HRQoL imaginable.

Defining the Utility of Consumption and Health and the MRS Between Consumption and Health

With this same general approach, we can define a utility ("value") function $V(C,H)$ as the utility created by different mixes of C and H, all within a fixed budget constraint.[5] We buy medical care to improve H, and what is left over from the fixed income is C. This makes it very clear that the "opportunity cost" of better H is foregone consumption, C.

To go further, we will make a slightly simplifying assumption to keep the intuition intact without getting buried in the math, namely that the utility function can be written as $V(C,H) = U(C)W(H)$. With this "setup," the utilities of C and H are "separable." Now the marginal utility of consumption is $U'(C)W(H)$ and the marginal utility of health is $U(C)W'(H)$.

Note that the marginal utility of consumption depends on the *level* of health, or more precisely, the utility derived from the level of health. As health shrinks, so does $W(H)$, and therefore the marginal utility of consumption shrinks. This is intuitively quite comfortable: The extra pleasure of a fancy restaurant dinner is lower if you have a headache, and lower yet (by far) if you are currently having kidney stone problems. The same is true for the marginal utility of health [it depends on $U(C)$], but when we keep C the same throughout this discussion, $U(C)$ does not vary, so the marginal utility of H varies only with the level of H—that is, only as $W'(H)$ varies.

Next, for small ("marginal") changes in C (dC) and H (dH), the change in overall happiness, $dV(C,H)$ is

$$dV(C,H) = U'(C)W(H)dC + U(C)W'(H)dH \qquad (2.1a)$$

Now comes a standard "trick": If we say, "Let's keep dV equal to zero as we shift around amounts of C and H," we are simply showing combinations of C and H that lead to the same level of utility—the economists' indifference curve similar to Figure 2.1, but now involving C and H

instead of $X1$ and $X2$. From this, when $dV(C,H) = 0$, we can easily derive the trade-off rate:

$$\frac{dC}{dH} = \frac{U(C)W'(H)}{U'(C)W(H)} \tag{2.1b}$$

In words, the "exchange rate," $\frac{dC}{dH}$, equals the ratio of the marginal utility of health in the numerator and the marginal utility of consumption in the denominator, all in the ex ante state, specifically $U'(C_0)W(H_0)$.

The Standard CEA Model

At this point, we come to a fork in the road. Following Yogi Berra's famous advice, we should take it.[6] But before we do, it is important to point out two assumptions in traditional CEA as formalized by Garber and Phelps (1997). The first assumption says that baseline health is "perfect," or more precisely, that $H_0 = 1$ (as we also have been assuming to this point). The second assumption is that the marginal utility of health, $W'(H)$, is constant, a crucial assumption, as we shall see momentarily.

There is a simple way to bring this into focus, by adding two new concepts. Define $\omega_C \equiv \dfrac{C_0 U'(C_0)}{U(C_0)}$, the elasticity of utility with respect to C, C_0 evaluated at baseline consumption, C_0, and similarly, $\omega_H \equiv \dfrac{H_0 W'(H_0)}{W(H_0)}$, the elasticity of utility with respect to H, also evaluated at H_0. These elasticities represent proportional rates of change in utility as either C or H change. Then Eq. (2.1b) shows the willingness to pay (WTP) for improved health—that is, the MRS between C and H. From this, it is readily apparent that

$$\text{WTP} \equiv \frac{dC}{dH_0} = \left[\frac{\omega_H}{\omega_C}\right]\left[\frac{C_0}{H_0}\right] \tag{2.2}$$

Traditional CEA and the practice thereof specify that both $\omega_H = 1$ and $H_0 = 1$, so the WTP measure (which we henceforth call K). With an implicit $H_0 = 1$ in the denominator, this sometimes is written as[7]

$$\text{WTP} \equiv K = \frac{C_0}{\omega_C} \tag{2.3}$$

Whenever this equation is shown, here or elsewhere, it contains the implicit $\left[\dfrac{1}{H_0}\right]$. Garber and Phelps (1997) arrived at this same point from a somewhat different direction, specifying that $K = \dfrac{U(C_0)}{U'(C_0)}$, which is equivalent to $K = \dfrac{C_0}{\omega_C}$ by using the definition for ω_C, where they omitted the implicit $\left[\dfrac{1}{H_0}\right]$.

This brings us to the specific novelty of GRACE. It relaxes these two restrictive assumptions, first allowing for $0 \le \omega_H \le 1$ and then, in Chapter 5 relating to permanent disability, the assumption that $H_0 = 1$.

It is again worth noting here that this definition of WTP clearly states that WTP is the utility of the foregone consumption necessary to "finance" the improved level of H, and Eq. (2.3) shows how that WTP rises as the utility of increasing C falls, all arising from declining marginal utility of C.

To highlight the consequences of the assumption of constant marginal utility, consider the following: If the same "non-diminishing returns" assumption was made about consumption of market goods and services (C)—that is, that $\omega_C = 1$—then WTP for a QALY would be 1 year's worth of C. WTP exceeds 1 year's worth of consumption (i.e., $K > C$) only with diminishing returns to C ($\omega_C < 1$). Because we can readily see that people are willing to pay more than a year's worth of income (or "consumption") for a 1-QALY gain in health, we know for sure that $\omega_C < 1$. We can expect similarly important consequences once we allow for $0 < \omega_H < 1$. The next section explores the consequences of relaxing the restrictive assumption that $\omega_H = 1$.

DIMINISHING RETURNS TO HEALTH

Willingness to Pay (WTP) in the GRACE model

Lakdawalla and Phelps (2020, 2021, 2022) introduce diminishing returns into the world of CEA, allowing the more-general (and realistic) assumption that $0 < \omega_H < 1$. This is the core concept of the GRACE model.

The generalization is both simple and important. Remember that Eq. (2.1a) analyzes the trade-off between C and H with "excellent" health $(H_0 = 1)$. We now consider a situation in which our representative consumer considers the trade-off between C and H *as if* an illness had occurred, driving down H to a lower level. We therefore now consider the trade-off rate not between H_0 and C but, rather, between H_{1S} and C, where H_{1S} is the level of untreated illness in a subsequent period ("period 1"). With diminishing marginal utility, this will be a different trade-off rate than the earlier comparison.

A useful way to think about this is to ask how much a consumer would pay for access to a treatment for an illness *in the next period* through an insurance premium that must be paid *in this period*. This makes it very clear that the trade-off is between current consumption (C) and health in the possible future sick state (H_{1S}). For a specific health benefit "B" from medical treatment in the next period, the total value of that treatment would be $\text{WTP} \times B \times p \times \phi$, where p is the probability of surviving into the next period, and ϕ is the probability the illness occurs, given survival. Ignoring for a moment these two probabilities, let's focus on the value trade-off. We can now rewrite Eq. (2.1a) to deal with this situation. The MRS is

$$\text{MRS} = U'(C)W(H_0)dC + U(C)W'(H_{1S})dH \qquad (2.4)$$

Note that we are still using $U'(C)W(H_0)$ to express the marginal utility of consumption. It continues to use the health level without sickness, H_0. However, the level of health used to evaluate the marginal utility of health has changed to the level of untreated sickness, so the marginal utility of health now equals $U(C)W'(H_{1S})$.

From this, we can derive an expression similar but not identical to Eq. (2.1b):

$$MRS = \frac{W'(H_{1s})U(C)}{U'(C)W(H_0)} \tag{2.5a}$$

Equation (2.5a) is *almost* identical to Eq. (2.1b). In fact, we can write Eq. (2.5a) as Eq. (2.1) with an extra "multiplier" stuck on the end:

$$MRS = \frac{W'(H_{1s})U(C)}{U'(C)W(H_0)} = \frac{W'(H_0)U(C)}{U'(C)W(H_0)}\left[\frac{W'(H_{1S})}{W'(H_0)}\right] \tag{2.5b}$$

Lakdawalla and Phelps (2020) define this new "appended" ratio as $R \equiv \frac{W'(H_{1S})}{W'(H_0)}$. (Technically, they define it as $R \equiv \frac{W'(E(H_{1S}))}{W'(H_0)}$, to allow for the possibility of stochastic health; we come to this generalization later.) It is the severity-of-illness adjustment made to WTP in the baseline state, which in turn is described in Eq. (2.1b). Because the marginal utility of H rises as H falls, then $W'(H_{1S}) > W'(H_0)$ so, necessarily, $R > 1$. As we shall see momentarily, R can be *much* larger than 1 for high-severity illnesses (low values of H_{1S}).

This leads to an important difference between standard CEA and GRACE. In GRACE, WTP for improved health care is greater for lower levels of untreated health than for the same health gain at better health: WTP grows with illness severity. In standard CEA, WTP is the same, no matter what the level of untreated illness severity. This is the first primary difference between standard CEA and GRACE.

Combining these changes leads to the modified WTP expression that is central to the GRACE methodology. Rather than the traditional WTP in Eq. (2.3), with a bit of algebraic manipulation, Eq. (2.5b) becomes

$$K_{\text{GRACE}} = \left[\frac{C_0}{H_0}\right]\left[\frac{\omega_H}{\omega_C}\right]R = K\omega_H R \tag{2.6}$$

In Eq. (2.6), the elasticity of utility with respect to H, ω_H, has been explicitly introduced (instead of implicitly assuming that it equals 1.0 at all times), and the new multiplier R has also been acknowledged. We will turn momentarily to ways to estimate R, but for now, we continue to focus on the diminishing returns to health, expressed by the level of ω_H. Recall that with positive but diminishing marginal utility of H, $0 < \omega_H < 1$.

In virtually all the health economics literature, with the exception of CEA, economists assume that there are diminishing returns to H, just as there are for C, and for all other economic "goods." Aristotle, cited at the beginning of this chapter, recognized this fact more than 2,000 years ago. The assumption that $\omega_H = 1$ is out of step with modern economic analysis and conflicts with real-world evidence. GRACE repairs that deficiency in the standard CEA model.[8]

Figure 2.2 shows how the "R effect" occurs. On the vertical axis is consumption (C) and on the horizontal axis the level of health (H). In "perfect" health, $H = H_0$, and when the illness occurs, $H = H_{1S}$. The slope is greater at H_{1S} than at H_0 because of diminishing returns to H. In other words, diminishing returns to health means that the same gain in H has more value to those who begin in worse health than people in "good" health. As a result, R will be systematically higher for severe illnesses compared to mild ones.

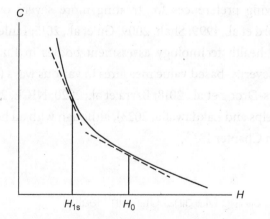

Figure 2.2 Indifference curve showing the marginal rate of substitution at two levels of H. As H declines, the marginal rate of substitution (slope of the tangent lines) increases.

The Preface gave several examples of diminishing returns to housing space, income, and vacation time. In health care, the same concept applies. If one could add 0.1 units of HRQoL to two otherwise identical people, would that health improvement create more value to a person beginning at HRQoL of 0.5 or 0.9? The answer is intuitively obvious; it would have greater value to the person with lower baseline health. In the presence of diminishing returns to health, the benefit increases with untreated illness severity. The mathematical formulation confirms this intuition. This is the underlying concept in the multiplier R—it is the ratio of the marginal utilities that a person would have in two different states of health, since $R = \dfrac{W'(H_{1S})}{W'(H_0)}$. The proper basis of comparison in all cases (the denominator) is the marginal utility of the person with "baseline" (pre-illness) health, H_0.

Introducing R into the WTP measure sharply diverges from the usual CEA mantra that "a QALY is a QALY . . . ." The simple and logical introduction of diminishing returns to health shows that the value of an incremental improvement in QALYs rises as illness severity increases. The "QALY is a QALY . . ." concept can no longer can be viewed as a valid statement about the proper way to measure the value of improving people's health.

This change brings the formal model into line with population-based studies showing preferences for treating more severe over less severe illnesses (Nord et al., 1999; Shah, 2009; Gu et al., 2015; Linley and Hughes, 2013). Some health technology assessment bodies in Europe have also introduced severity-based value measures in various ways (Ottersen et al., 2016; Reckers-Droog et al., 2018; Barra et al., 2020; NICE, 2022; Skedgel et al., 2022; Phelps and Lakdawalla, 2023), although with ad hoc methods, as we discuss in Chapter 12.

Effects of Declining Marginal Utility in Health

In addition to the introduction of the R multiplier, we now consider the effects of declining marginal utility of health on K_{GRACE}. Since $0 < \omega_H \leq 1$,

$\left[\dfrac{\omega_H}{\omega_C}\right] \leq \left[\dfrac{1}{\omega_C}\right]$. This means that (before the severity of illness adjustment R is made), WTP is lower in the GRACE framework than in the traditional framework.

The logic is quite simple. In the standard formulation (see Eq. 2.3), WTP for improved health is the MRS "trade-off," which grows as the cost (in utility terms) of foregone consumption shrinks. This occurs because of the diminishing returns to C. The smaller is ω_C (i.e., the less utility loss that occurs as C shrinks), the greater is K.

The introduction of $\omega_H < 1$ does the same thing with regard to the way value changes as H itself changes. The smaller is ω_H, the smaller is WTP. This change simply makes the treatment of C and H symmetric in our understanding of the opportunity cost of improved health. Now, both for C and H, we have assumed diminishing marginal utility.

Adding Risk and Uncertain Health Outcomes

Thus far, we have calculated the value of health improvement under the assumption that people purchase insurance when healthy and can perfectly forecast their post-treatment health status in the future. This assumption is not very realistic, nor is it compatible with our focus on diminishing returns. Consumers with diminishing returns to utility over health improvement will also dislike bearing risk over their health. Assuming away all this uncertainty is sure to distort estimates of value for such consumers.

To address this problem, Lakdawalla and Phelps (2020, 2021, 2022) allow health in the sick state, H_{1S}, to be a random variable. To avoid the confusion associated with a random WTP for health, they evaluate WTP at the average sick state health level, defined as $\mu_H \equiv E(H_{1S})$, the expected value of the random variable, H_{1S}, for any particular illness event. As a result, the precise definition of R is given by $R \equiv \dfrac{W'(\mu_H)}{W'(H_0)}$.

In order to fully evaluate R, we must overcome the difficulty of estimating the health-related utility function, W. In general, economists view utility as difficult to observe and measure. Fortunately, the economic literature on risk preferences comes to our rescue. Lakdawalla and Phelps (2020, 2021, 2022) show how to measure the ratio R, based on measures of risk aversion in health and severity of illness (ℓ^*). We turn next to the tasks of estimating these key parameters.

Measurement of Illness Severity

Our new severity index, ℓ^*, is measured on a $[0, 1]$ scale, where $1 = $ "ideal" health and $0 = $ "worst health-related HRQoL imaginable." Again, we remind the reader that ℓ^* is an index of *health status*, not the utility of health. Define H_0 as the baseline level of health, commonly set so that $H_0 = 1$. Then, when μ_H is defined as the average level of untreated health (hence smaller than $H_0 = 1$), it follows that $\ell^* = \dfrac{H_0 - \mu_H}{H_0}$. We use this index of health loss to estimate R. But first, we need to take a small side excursion into the economics of risk.

Measurement of Attitudes Toward Risk

Economists commonly think about the level of risk aversion relating to financial risk, generally discussed in terms of how much people are willing to pay to remove financial risk. The entire insurance industry rests on the presence of risk aversion; without it, no rational person would buy insurance. The concept of risk aversion was formally developed by Pratt (1964) and Arrow (1971).

Relative risk aversion measures the income elasticity of the marginal utility of income. This measures how rapidly $U'(C)$ changes as C changes.[9] Assuming declining marginal utility of income, so that $U''(C) < 0$, relative risk aversion is

$$r_C^* = -C \frac{U''(C)}{U'(C)} > 0 \qquad\qquad (2.7a)$$

One can readily interpret r_C^* as the "income elasticity of the marginal utility of income." It proportionately assesses how fast *marginal* utility changes as C changes.

Subsequently, Kimball (1990) and others extended this concept to higher order derivatives of the utility function—relative prudence and relative temperance:

$$\pi^* = -C\left(\frac{U'''(C)}{U''(C)}\right) \tag{2.7b}$$

$$\tau^* = -C\left(\frac{U''''(C)}{U'''(C)}\right) \tag{2.7c}$$

Just as r_C^* describes how rapidly the marginal utility of income changes as C changes, relative prudence, π_C^*, describes how rapidly relative risk aversion, r_C^*, changes with C. Similarly, relative temperance, τ_C^*, describes how rapidly relative prudence, π_C^*, changes with C.[10] These parameters have a simple relationship between them when utility has constant relative risk aversion (CRRA), a common assumption in economic theory. In this case, $\pi_C^* = r_C^* + 1, \tau_C^* = r_C^* + 2, \ldots$ etc. If utility is expressed as the logarithm of C, so that $U(C) = ln(C)$, then $r_C^* = 1, \pi_C^* = 2, \tau_C^* = 3, \ldots$.

Combining Severity of Illness and Risk Attitudes

Two paths exist to determining R. The first method assumes that an exact representation of the utility function for $W(H)$ exists. For example, it might be assumed that $W(H)$ has the form of a constant elasticity of utility with respect to health, and the appropriate parameter (or parameters, in more general utility functions) has been properly estimated. From this, estimation of R is straightforward.

For example, suppose that $W(H)$ has the form of CRRA, where ω_H is constant over all levels of H. Then, $W(H) = H^\gamma$, and marginal utility is $W'(H) = \frac{\gamma}{H^{1-\gamma}}$, so R can be derived by evaluating this expression at $H = E(H_{1S}) = \mu_H$ and at $H = H_0 = 1$ and then taking their ratio. Then,

$R = \dfrac{1^{1-\gamma}}{\mu_H^{1-\gamma}} = \dfrac{1}{\mu_H^{1-\gamma}}$. Now assume that $\gamma = 0.4$, so that $R = \dfrac{1}{\mu_H^{0.6}}$. If the un-

treated sick state has an average level of health of $\mu_H = 0.8$, a relatively

mild illness, then $R = \dfrac{1}{.8745} = 1.14$. For a moderately severe illness where

$\mu_H = 0.5$, $R = \dfrac{1}{.6598} = 1.516$. For a very severe illness, where $\mu_H = 0.1$,

$R = \dfrac{1}{0.1^{0.6}} = \dfrac{1}{.2511} = 3.98$. The value of R grows as the power param-

eter grows. If $\gamma = 0.9$, for the same illness levels (serially), $R = 1.22$, then
$R = 1.87$, and for the most severe illness, $R = 7.94$.

The same can be readily done for any exact utility function that has
been assumed. However, if analysts prefer to avoid specifying an exact
utility function, then an alternative exists, using the Taylor series expansion of the ratio of marginal utilities, which we discuss next.

The new relative risk preferences in the previous section provide
the basis for measuring the severity ratio R simply, once people's risk
preferences regarding H are estimated. This process provides a solution for *any* sufficiently differentiable utility function in H. To do this,
Lakdawalla and Phelps (2020) introduced comparable measures of relative risk preferences over the domain of health. As with consumption,

$$r_H^* = -H\left(\frac{W''(H)}{W'(H)}\right) \text{ describes relative risk aversion with respect to } H \quad (2.8a)$$

$$\pi_H^* = -H\left(\frac{W'''(H)}{W''(H)}\right) \text{ describes how rapidly } r_H^* \text{ changes with } H \quad (2.8b)$$

$$\tau_H^* = -H\left(\frac{W''''(H)}{W'''(H)}\right) \text{ describes how rapidly } \pi_H^* \text{ changes with } H \quad (2.8c)$$

Taken together, and using the standard mathematical tool of Taylor series
expansions,[11] Lakdawalla and Phelps (2020) proved that we can estimate R

using these risk-preference parameters and the average severity-of-illness measure for any disorder, $\ell^* = \dfrac{H_0 - \mu_H}{H_0}$:

$$R = 1 + \frac{r_H^* \ell^*}{1!} + \frac{1}{2!} r_H^* \pi_H^* \ell^{*2} + \frac{1}{3!} r_H^* \pi_H^* \tau_H^* \ell^{*3} + \dots \qquad (2.9)$$

Note that $R = 1$ either if there is no risk aversion (r_H^* and higher terms equal zero) or if health losses (ℓ^*) equal zero.

At this point, a (fairly plausible) simplification greatly aids intuition and understanding—the assumption of CRRA. With that simplifying assumption, $\pi_C^* = r_C^* + 1, \tau_C^* = r_C^* + 2, \dots$etc. Then Table 2.1 shows how R grows as the severity of untreated illness grows, and that growth rate is larger when r_H^* is larger.[12]

We'll return to Table 2.1 several times, so you might wish to "flag" this page somehow.

Average R Score for Nonmarginal Changes in H

While we have made clear that R represents the *marginal* value of improving HRQoL, we have not yet dealt with the question of how to value large, nonmarginal changes in HRQoL. In this section, we provide the basis for accomplishing this task. In traditional CEA, this is not an issue because marginal benefit equals average benefit. In GRACE, that no longer holds, and we must deal with this issue through further analysis. This is yet another consequences of how valuation of medical treatments changes when "a QALY is a QALY . . ." no longer holds. For treatments producing large gains in health (measured by large reductions in ℓ^*), the marginal value of the first "smidgen" of health improvement gets valued as specified in the relevant cell in Table 2.1. But once that small increment in health is achieved, the "next" incremental gain in HRQoL has a slightly lower value. We need the average value across the health gain, rather than

Table 2.1 R as Function of r_H^* and ℓ^*

r_H^*	Severity (ℓ^*)									
	0	0.1	0.2	0.3	0.4	0.5	0.6	0.7	0.8	0.9
0	1	1	1	1	1	1	1	1	1	1
0.1	1	1.01	1.02	1.04	1.05	1.07	1.1	1.13	1.17	1.26
0.2	1	1.02	1.05	1.07	1.11	1.15	1.2	1.27	1.38	1.57
0.3	1	1.03	1.07	1.12	1.17	1.21	1.32	1.44	1.62	1.99
0.4	1	1.04	1.09	1.15	1.22	1.32	1.43	1.62	1.9	2.5
0.5	1	1.05	1.12	1.2	1.29	1.41	1.58	1.83	2.24	3.16
0.6	1	1.07	1.14	1.24	1.36	1.52	1.73	2.06	2.62	3.98
0.7	1	1.08	1.17	1.28	1.43	1.62	1.9	2.32	3.08	5.01
0.8	1	1.09	1.2	1.33	1.5	1.74	2.08	2.62	3.62	6.35
0.9	1	1.1	1.22	1.38	1.58	1.87	2.28	2.96	4.27	7.94
1.0	1	1.26	1.25	1.43	1.67	2	2.5	3.33	5	10

using the marginal gain at the level of untreated health, to measure the value of large, nonmarginal changes in HRQoL. Two methods are available to complete this task—numerical integration and a Taylor series approximation to the actual integral. We discuss each in turn.

Numerical Integration

Numerical integration provides one well-established way to approximate this sum of marginal gains. This method estimates the total value by adding up the area of a series of rectangles of area that "fill up" the area under the curve, in our case the curve being the graph of $R = f(\ell^*)$. Obviously, this type of approximation is increasingly accurate as the width of each rectangle narrows.[13]

Table 2.1 gives the marginal values of R for values of ℓ^* in intervals of width 0.1. We can imagine (and could potentially estimate) a function stating that $R = f(\ell^*)$ and graph it as a continuous curve. Then the relevant area under that curve would give the total value of a nonmarginal treatment. Rather than undertaking that task, we can use the specific values of R to estimate the area under that hypothetical curve by using the trapezoidal method of numerical integration, which states that the area under the $R = f(\ell^*)$ function is approximated by the sum of a series of rectangles, each with width Δ.

$$\sum_{a=H_0(1-\ell^*)}^{H_0(1-\ell^*+\mu_B)} \left[\int_a^{a+\Delta} f(\ell^*)d\ell^* \right] \approx \sum_{a=H_0(1-\ell^*)}^{H_0(1-\ell^*+\mu_B)} \left[\Delta \frac{[f(a+\Delta)+f(a)]}{2} \right] \qquad (2.10)$$

In words, Eq. (2.10) simply adds up a sequence of rectangles of width Δ, where the height of each rectangle is the average of the height at each of its sides, as determined by the values of R at each side. The summations run from $H_0(1-\ell^*)$, the level of HRQoL before treatment, to $H_0(1-\ell^*+\mu_B)$, the level of HRQoL after treatment.

This approximation is exact when $f(\ell^*)$ is linear but overstates the true value when $R = f(\ell^*)$ is convex, with the magnitude of overstatement rising as the width Δ increases. Figure 2.3 illuminates this issue. The left-hand panel shows a linear version of $R = f(\ell^*)$. The shaded bar represents the rectangle used by the trapezoidal method. The bar's height is the average of the two "boundary" values of $R = f(\ell^*)$ in the interval. This rectangle omits the area B but includes area A in the approximation. When $f(\ell^*)$ is linear, these areas are equal, and the approximation is exact.

The right-hand panel of Figure 2.3 shows the situation when $R = f(\ell^*)$ is convex (as is true in our case). Here, because the rectangle has fixed and finite (not infinitesimal) width, the omitted area under the curve, B, has a smaller area than area A, which should not be included when calculating the area under the curve, so the approximation overstates the true value. The wider is each rectangle, the greater the error.

In our approximation, $\Delta = 0.1$ (because those are the intervals in Table 2.1), and $\frac{[f(a+\Delta)+f(a)]}{2}$ represents the average R value measured at the right and left edges of each rectangle. Thus, for example, when $r_H^* = 0$, the upper-right-hand corner cell of Table 2.2 and its next-adjacent value to the left are both $R = 1$, so the average value of R for the two sides of the rectangle in Table 2.2 is exactly 1.0. With an interval width of 0.1, when $r_H^* = 0$ (row 1 of Table 2.2, representing standard CEA methods), each increment

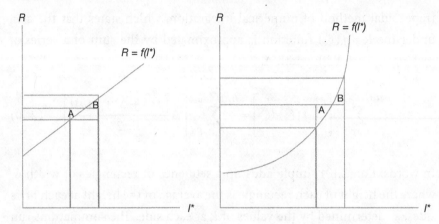

Figure 2.3 Illustration of the trapezoidal numerical integration with a linear function (*left*) and convex function (*right*). With convex functions, this approach can slightly overestimate the area under the curve, with the magnitude of error rising as the width of the rectangles rises.

adds 0.1 to HRQoL. Adding up across row 1, a cure from $\ell^* = 0.9$ nets a total of 0.9 HRQoL increase.

Table 2.2 shows these cumulative values, not only for $r_H^* = 0$ (the top row) but also for incrementally increasing values of r_H^* up to 1. To further understand how Table 2.2 is constructed, in the bottom row ($r_H^* = 1$) of Table 2.1, the average height (R value) of the last rectangle is 7.5 (the average of 10 and 5), and the width is 0.1 for each rectangle, so the first improvement in HRQoL from $\ell^* = 0.9$ to 0.8 adds 0.75 HRQoL units to the total gain. The next rectangle in the summation has an average height of 4.166 . . . (averaging 5.0 and 3.33 . . .), thus adding 0.417 HRQoL units to the total. A complete cure, adding across the entire row, would yield the 2.39 HRQoL units, the sum across the entire row in Table 2.1, as shown in the lower right-hand corner of Table 2.2.

Recall that a "complete cure" in our discussions increases HRQoL by 0.9 HRQoL units. Turning to treatments that provide less than a full cure, when $r_H^* = 0$, the patient gains 0.1 HRQoL units in value for each improvement of 0.1 in the illness severity index, ℓ^*. If we improve HRQoL from 0.9 to 0.5, the gain is the difference between the two values in the appropriate row for r_H^*. When $r_H^* = 0$, that difference is 0.9 − 0.5 = 0.4 HRQoL units.

These values, when $r_H^* = 0$ are proper only when there are constant returns to HRQoL, and therefore "a QALY is a QALY . . . ."

Now perform the same calculations when $r_H^* = 0.5$. A complete cure from a starting point of $\ell^* = 0.9$ gains 1.38 HRQoL units, and an improvement in HRQoL from $\ell^* = 0.9$ to $\ell^* = 0.5$ gains $1.38 - 0.59 = 0.79$ HRQoL units.

Finally, when $r_H^* = 1$, a complete cure is worth 2.39 HRQoL units (not 0.9 as would be measured in standard CEA), and a gain from $\ell^* = .09$ to $\ell^* = .05$ is worth 1.68 HRQoL units $(2.39 - 0.71)$, not the 0.4 HRQoL units when $r_H^* = 0$, which represents the value for standard CEA.

Table 2.2 again highlights how GRACE refutes the notion that "a QALY is a QALY is a QALY . . . ." As r_H^* rises, the gains from the same increment in HRQoL rise exponentially.

Table 2.2 also highlights that the distinction between GRACE and standard CEA methods is small for low levels of illness severity—for example, $\ell^* \leq 0.2$—particularly when coupled with low values for r_H^*. For these illness levels, the degree of risk aversion in HRQoL, r_H^*, has minimal influence on the value metrics. But as illness severity rises, the importance of knowing the proper degree of risk aversion increases rapidly.

Integration of Taylor Series Approximation to R

An alternative approach to calculating the average value would use the integral of the Taylor series expansion directly and then evaluate it at the appropriate values (the highest and lowest values of ℓ^* that describe the

Table 2.2 Cumulative Value of QALY Gains for Various Values of r_H^*

r_H^*	Degree of Disability (ℓ^*)								
	0.1	0.2	0.3	0.4	0.5	0.6	0.7	0.8	0.9
0	0.10	0.20	0.30	0.40	0.50	0.60	0.70	0.80	0.90
0.1	0.10	0.20	0.31	0.41	0.52	0.62	0.74	0.85	0.97
0.3	0.10	0.21	0.32	0.43	0.56	0.69	0.83	0.98	1.16
0.5	0.10	0.21	0.33	0.45	0.59	0.74	0.91	1.11	1.38
0.7	0.10	0.22	0.34	0.47	0.63	0.80	1.01	1.28	1.69
0.9	0.11	0.22	0.35	0.50	0.67	0.88	1.14	1.50	2.11
1	0.11	0.24	0.37	0.53	0.71	0.94	1.23	1.64	2.39

nonmarginal change in health from a medical intervention). Since the Taylor series formula for R is given as

$$R = 1 + \frac{r_H^* \ell^*}{1!} + \frac{1}{2!} r_H^* \pi_H^* \ell^{*2} + \frac{1}{3!} r_H^* \pi_H^* \tau_H^* \ell^{*3} + \dots \qquad (2.11a)$$

then the integral is

$$\int_a^b R(\ell^*) d\ell^* = \ell^* \left[1 + \frac{r_H^* \ell^*}{2!} + \frac{1}{3!} r_H^* \pi_H^* \ell^{*2} + \frac{1}{4!} r_H^* \pi_H^* \tau_H^* \ell^{*3} + \dots \right] \qquad (2.11b)$$

where a and b (respectively) are the lowest and highest values of ℓ^* involved in a specific treatment. This requires knowing the risk parameters to calculate, of course. For example, suppose that utility in health is CRRA and $r^* = 0.8$, so $\pi^* = 1.8$ and $\tau^* = 2.8, \dots$. Then the value of the integral from a to b is as follows:[14]

$$\int_a^b R(\ell^*) d\ell^* = \ell^* \left[1 + + \frac{1}{2!}(0.8)\ell^* + \frac{1}{3!}(0.8*1.8)\ell^{*2} + \frac{1}{4!}(0.8*1.8*2.8)\ell^{*3} + \dots \right.$$

$$(2.11c)$$

To continue the example, if the treatment shifts ℓ^* from 0.6 to 0.1, a substantial improvement of 0.5 HRQoL units, the marginal values of R at the end points are 2.08 and 1.09 respectively, and integral under the R curve is 0.733. The average R score is 0.733/0.5 = 1.47. If the same technology was valued using standard CEA methods, the added value would be 0.5 QALYs at an average R score of 1.0. Therefore, the GRACE method imputes a value that is approximately 50% larger for this particular intervention that standard CEA would allow. Note that the average of the two boundary scores (1.58) would overstate the QALY gain because of the curvature of the R function.

Obviously, the average value increases as the beginning severity level (b) increases. If the same 0.5 QALY gain began at a severity level of $\ell^* = 0.8$, the R values at the end points would be 1.33 and 3.62, and the integral under the R curve is 1.032, for an average value of 2.06. Again, note that the average of the boundary values of the integral (2.47) overstates the true integral, this time even more, because the evaluation takes place at a steeper section of the R curve.

One cautionary note for using this method is that the Taylor series expansion does not converge very rapidly for larger values of ℓ^*, so the estimated integral must be extended well past the terms shown in Eq. (2.11b). Chapter 8 provides methods to do this by building from estimates of r_H^* using a specific utility function (hyperbolic absolute risk aversion [HARA]) that has widespread use in economic theory.[15]

Combining Decreasing Returns (ω_H) and Severity of Illness (R)

The combination of the first two changes created by GRACE—declining marginal utility (ω_H) and the risk adjustment factor R—leads directly to two important observations. First, compared with traditional CEA measures of WTP, GRACE leads to *lower* WTP for low-severity illnesses and *higher* WTP for more severe illnesses. GRACE "taketh away" WTP for low-severity disease treatments and "giveth" more for high-severity disease treatments.

Some people seem to forget this part of GRACE and express concerns that using GRACE value measures to set medical care prices will increase long-terms medical spending because of the severity multiplier factor R. Chapter 11 demonstrates when this is true, and when not true, using various examples.

A Note About Increasing Returns to Health

The discussion above presumes diminishing marginal utility from health, but GRACE is even more flexible than this. Simply stated, GRACE removes the restriction that marginal utility from health is constant. Thus, it accommodates the possibility that marginal utility from health is rising over certain regions; for instance, patients may exhibit rising marginal utility of health in very severe health states, as suggested by the "value of hope" concept (Lakdawalla et al., 2012). GRACE continues to be useful even when marginal utility from health is rising. While the formulae remain unchanged, one caveat emerges: Taylor series approximations can become less reliable in regions where the utility of health switches from concave to convex or vice versa. In these circumstances, analysts will be better served by estimating the underlying utility function, $W(H)$, and computing exact (rather than approximate) values for GRACE. We present the complete exact estimation approach to estimating the full GRACE model in Appendix 6.1.

SUMMARY

Introducing diminishing returns to health in the utility function of a rational decision-maker markedly changes the proper way to value medical interventions. In this chapter, we have shown how this one simple assumption reduces the value of interventions that treat low-severity illnesses but (through the illness severity multiplier R) raise the value of treatments of high-severity illnesses, all compared with traditional CEA models.

The concept of diminishing returns brings with it a parallel concept—risk aversion. They spring from the same notion. With diminishing returns, increases and decreases in wealth (or health) of equal amount do not have the same utility value. Increases are worth less, and declines are more "painful" in terms of lost utility. This leads to formal methods to analyze risk and peoples' aversion to it. In Chapter 3, we explore the important concept of risk aversion in the level of health and its consequences for valuing medical interventions.

How Uncertain Treatment Outcomes Affect Value

The special economic problems of medical care can be explained
as adaptations to the existence of uncertainty in the incidence of
disease and the efficacy of treatment.

—Kenneth J. Arrow (1963)

THE INTUITION

The History of Risk Reduction

People generally do not like risky outcomes. The existence of extensive insurance markets in almost every society in the world attests to this. Hindu
writings discuss insurance mechanisms dating to the 3rd century BCE.
Chinese merchants diversified their risk by using multiple sailing ships to
carry cargo that could have been sent on one vessel. This simple method
of "self-insurance" reduced risk at the added cost of using multiple ships
to move the same amount of cargo.

The first written description of a formal insurance arrangement appears
in the famous Code of Hammurabi, circa 1750 BCE. Literally written in
stone, the Code of Hammurabi says that merchants, for an extra fee on

Valuing Health. Charles E. Phelps and Darius N. Lakdawalla, Oxford University Press. © Oxford University Press 2024.
DOI: 10.1093/oso/9780197686287.003.0003

their loan to support a trade expedition, could buy relief from having to repay the loan if the ship was lost at sea. Thus, the lender also became an insurer.

The concept of insurance became intertwined with that of "usury" in medieval Europe, which was frowned on by religious authorities, but the concept of insurance nevertheless emerged triumphant. As a famous example, the King of Portugal, in 1293 CE, established by common agreement among ship owners a formal maritime insurance plan. By the 1700s, insurance became deeply institutionalized, most strongly in London, England. The most famous of such institutions, Lloyds of London, founded by Edward Lloyd in 1688, still persists today, with a reputation that almost any type of risk can be covered through the Lloyds network. This now includes risks of space flight and deep submarine diving.

There are counterexamples, of course. The entire gambling industry poses a challenge to economists' standard view that consumers do not like risky events. When people gamble, they reveal a preference for risky over non-risky alternatives. The field of behavioral economics focuses on such issues using prospect theory, which differs in significant ways from the standard expected utility theory that is the mainstay of economic analysis about risk. Our development of the generalized risk-adjusted cost-effectiveness (GRACE) model follows the standard economic model directly, and it may require subsequent modification as economists gain better understanding about peoples' overall attitudes toward risk.

Treatment Options with Differing Risk

Our "problem" concerns how people view risky outcomes regarding their health and, in particular, risks relating to health-related quality of life (HRQoL). Several potential situations arise, all supposing that you have a very painful knee joint from permanent athletic damage and a constant and persistent HRQoL of 0.6 on a scale from 0 to 1. You are offered a new therapy with the following outcome possibilities:

Treatment A

HRQoL = 0.9 with probability 0.5
HRQoL = 0.3 with probability 0.5

Doing nothing (i.e., declining to use Treatment A) leaves you with a HRQoL level of 0.6. Accepting Treatment A has an expected HRQoL level of 0.6 but both a potential high-benefit outcome and an equal chance of making your situation much worse (permanently). Treatment A gives you equal chances of a 0.3 boost in HRQoL and a 0.3 loss in HRQoL. Standard cost-effectiveness analysis (CEA) models treat these two choices as equivalent because both have an expected outcome of 0.6 HRQoL. It says that consumers would be indifferent between Treatment A and "doing nothing." Which would you prefer? If you answered "do nothing," you are either risk averse or risk neutral. If you answered Treatment A, you are risk preferring.

Now consider the same initial situation, but add two additional choices:

Treatment B

HRQoL = 0.8 with probability 1

Treatment C

HRQoL = 1 with probability 0.3 (perfect health)
HRQoL = 0.8 with probability 0.4
HRQoL = 0.6 with probability 0.3 (no improvement)

Both Treatment B and Treatment C have an expected outcome of 0.8 HRQoL units, a gain of 0.2 HRQoL units per year for your remaining lifetime. In any model of rational decision-making, Treatments B and C are preferred to Treatment A, but standard CEA models consider Treatments B and C equivalent because they have the same expected outcome. Which would you prefer? If you are risk averse, you should prefer Treatment B, avoiding the uncertainty of Treatment C.

Now consider still another alternative:

Treatment D

HRQoL = 1 with probability 0.2
HRQoL = 0.75 with probability 0.8

As with Treatments B and C, Treatment D has an expected outcome of 0.8 HRQoL units. With Treatment D, compared with Treatment B, you give up a bit of expected HRQoL units 80 percent of the time, in exchange for a 20 percent chance of a perfect cure. Treatment D has a positively skewed distribution of treatment outcomes. Which would you prefer? Here, the "right answer," even for risk-averse persons, is not necessarily determined.

The GRACE method of valuing medical interventions accounts for variance and skewness of the distribution of treatment outcomes. More variance is "bad," and GRACE predicts that risk-averse people will prefer Treatment B to Treatment C because Treatment C has greater variability and the distribution around the mean is symmetric.

In GRACE, more positive skewness is an economic "good." It provides a value of hope for a perfect cure (in this example). The distribution of Treatment D is positively skewed. The chances of a very positive outcome are increased, with very little "downside" potential in exchange. GRACE states that some people could well prefer Treatment D to Treatment B (or, of course, Treatment C), depending on their particular attitudes toward risk. The next section describes the mathematical model that helps sort out these types of issues.

THE MATH

The underlying concept involves the distinction that people do not value risky outcomes as much as they value certain outcomes with the same average value. That is, the expected utility of a treatment with random benefit is less than the expected utility of a similar treatment with no variability. In mathematical terms, where H_s^T is the stochastic post-treatment health value, and H_s^U is the stochastic untreated health level of any given disease or injury, the expected utility depends on the change in the risk profile in the treated state compared with the untreated state. If the utility function is known exactly—for example, constant relative risk aversion (CRRA) utility, as discussed in Chapter 2—then by combining the distribution of health outcomes in the treated and untreated states and an exact utility function, analysts can estimate $E(W(H_S^T))$ and $E(W(H_S^U))$ directly. Appendix 6.1 provides more details on this approach in the general multiperiod setting. However, if analysts do not wish to assume an exact functional form for utility, then a Taylor series expansion method can again be used. The next section discusses this approach in detail.

Risk Aversion and How It Applies to Uncertain Treatment Outcomes

In Chapter 2, we introduced the concept of declining marginal utility of HRQoL, a phenomenon summarized by the elasticity of utility with respect to H, ω_H. We also noted that this idea closely relates to the concept of risk aversion—the dislike of uncertain outcomes. Virtually all earlier economic analysis regarding risk aversion has focused on how financial uncertainty affects value of various risky investments or income streams. One relevant summary measure of this is the relative risk aversion measure, $r_C^* = -C\dfrac{U''(C)}{U'(C)}$. It measures how fast the marginal utility of consumption changes as C itself changes.[1] An extensive survey of the economic literature concluded that ". . . relative risk aversion is larger than but near one, and slightly increasing or constant." (Meyer and Meyer, 2005, p. 245). The GRACE method introduces the parallel concept of risk aversion in HRQoL: $r_H^* = -H\dfrac{W''(H)}{W'(H)}$. It simply measures how fast the marginal utility of health declines as H increases.

As with consumption, C, the concepts of diminishing marginal utility (ω_H) and risk aversion (r_H^*) are closely linked.[2] When utility in H has

CRRA, then $\omega_H + r_H^* = 1$. Because positive but declining marginal utility in health requires that $0 < \omega_H < 1$, it naturally follows that when utility is CRRA, $r_H^* < 1$. As the discussion in Chapter 2 (surrounding Table 2.3) notes, however, if utility is decreasing relative risk aversion or increasing relative risk aversion, this tight link can be broken, and values of $r_H^* > 1$ are possible.

Standard health technology assessment (HTA) practice routinely reports the *average* difference in HRQoL outcomes between new medical treatments (T) and the relevant comparison treatment (C). Lakdawalla and Phelps (2020) call this difference μ_B, where B stands for treatment benefit. If people are not risk averse in HRQoL, then this measure suffices when comparing medical interventions. However, if real people are risk averse in H, then μ_B no longer provides a sufficient measure of differences between alternative medical interventions.

Measuring the Effects of Uncertain Treatment Outcomes

We now reach the position where we want to quantify the importance of uncertainty in treatment outcomes on value of medical interventions. At this point, it should come as no surprise to the reader that the solution to this problem involves statistical measures beyond means—variances, skewness, and possibly kurtosis—and the associated risk preference parameters, relative risk aversion (r_H^*), relative prudence (π_H^*), and (if feasible) relative temperance (τ_H^*) that measure risk preferences in the domain of HRQoL (H).

Once again, the pioneering British mathematician Brook Taylor comes to the rescue: We can express the effects of variability of treatment outcomes using a Taylor series expansion that provides an estimate of the value of *any* sufficiently differentiable utility function. With the reminder of the definitions of the relative risk parameters (see Chapter 2, Eqs. 2.8a–2.8c), Lakdawalla and Phelps (2020) proved that the proper adjustment for risk is to multiply the average gain in HRQoL by this complicated-looking factor:

$$\varepsilon \approx 1+\left[\frac{\mu_H}{\mu_B}\right]\left[\begin{array}{c}-\frac{1}{2}r_H^*\left(\frac{1}{\mu_H}\right)^2\Delta\sigma_H^2+\frac{1}{6}\pi_H^*r_H^*\left(\frac{1}{\mu_H}\right)^3\Delta\left[\gamma_1\sigma_H^3\right]\\-\frac{1}{24}\tau_H^*\pi_H^*r_H^*\left(\frac{1}{\mu_H}\right)^4\Delta\left[\gamma_2\sigma_H^4\right]\cdots\end{array}\right] \quad (3.1)$$

The "approximately equal" condition comes from not including higher order risk terms beyond the fourth-order Taylor series term, involving kurtosis of the distributions of risk.[3] Even that term may be difficult to estimate in real-world clinical trials, and the approximation may end with the third-order term involving $\Delta[\gamma_1\sigma_H^3]$.

Let's parse out this complicated-looking formula one piece at a time. Start with the first term, involving relative risk aversion: $-\frac{1}{2}r_H^*\left(\frac{1}{\mu_H}\right)^2\Delta\sigma_H^2$.

The $\Delta\sigma_H^2$ term is simply the *difference* in the variances of the outcomes for the treatment (T) and comparison (C) therapies. This difference gets "normalized" by the average health outcome in the untreated state, the term $\left(\frac{1}{\mu_H}\right)^2$. This makes the "difference in variance" term just like the common coefficient of variation, except that the numerator is the *change* in variances. Finally, these get multiplied by $\left(-\frac{1}{2}r_H^*\right)$. This is simply the standard "risk premium" multiplier from the world of financial economics translated into uncertainty in health outcomes.[4] Relative risk aversion, r_H^*, is positive. This means that technologies that *reduce* variability of outcomes (so that $\Delta\sigma_H^2 < 0$) *add* value beyond the average gain, μ_B. The reverse is true, of course, if the technology adds variability to HRQoL outcomes. We call this "the value of insurance." It reflects the value of a medical intervention in terms of reduced uncertainty of outcomes.

In addition to this, of course, there is reduced financial uncertainty that comes with reduced variance in health outcomes. Without knowing the health insurance coverage of the affected individual, we do not know how that plays out, so we ignore it here. For our purposes, it is as if we assume that the patients whom we analyze have full-coverage insurance, so they have no concerns about financial variability. To see how that problem is solved, see Phelps (2022a), which assesses demand for insurance separately, but using similar (Taylor series) methods to those we use here.

The next term, $\frac{1}{6}\pi_H^* r_H^* \left(\frac{1}{\mu_H}\right)^3 \Delta\left[\gamma_1 \sigma_H^3\right]$, does the same thing as the variance term, except that it deals with changes in the positive skewness of the distribution of outcomes, $\Delta\left[\gamma_1 \sigma_H^3\right]$. Here, γ_1 is the Pearson skewness coefficient, and $\sigma_H^3 = \left(\sigma_H^2\right)^{\frac{3}{2}}$. The Pearson skewness coefficient, γ_1, equals zero in symmetric distributions (e.g., the normal distribution). The value $\gamma_1 \sigma_H^3$ must be computed separately for both the T and C populations, and then the difference of those two values becomes $\Delta[\gamma_1 \sigma_H^3]$. That difference is then normalized (as before) by $\left(\frac{1}{\mu_H}\right)^3$. Then that product is multiplied by $\frac{1}{6}\pi_H^* r_H^*$.[5] Once more, r_H^* is relative risk aversion in HRQoL and π_H^* is relative prudence, the magnitude of which tells us how fast r_H^* changes with H.[6]

We call this the "value of hope." For any given degree of variance in a distribution of health outcomes, more positive skewness is an economic "good" because it increases the chances of a very favorable outcome. Thus, independent of the changes in variance, technologies that increase positive skewness (thereby increasing the chances of a very favorable outcomes) add value beyond the mean difference in outcomes. There is also added value from reducing negative skewness, the situation in which treatment outcomes are skewed toward highly unfavorable outcomes. Thus, the value of hope also contains what we might call the "value of assurance" that terrible outcomes are less likely to occur, given any specific variance in the outcomes.

GRACE provides a formal way to incorporate both the value of insurance and the value of hope into a unified model, as sought by the ISPOR economic task force to provide a comprehensive measure value (Lakdawalla et al., 2018). That report expressed concern that adding these two components to the value measure might lead to "double counting" in some way. Equation (3.1) provides a formal way to incorporate both of these "values" while ensuring that there is no double counting.

The final term in Eq. (3.1) is $-\frac{1}{24}\tau_H^* \pi_H^* r_H^* \left(\frac{1}{\mu_H}\right)^2 \Delta\left[\gamma_2 \sigma_H^4\right]$. This is just like the previous terms except that it deals with changes in kurtosis of the distribution of outcomes.[7] Kurtosis measures how "fat" the tails are in the distribution, so greater kurtosis magnifies the effects of variance. Thus (because of the minus sign in the term), shrinking kurtosis provides a separate economic benefit. As noted previously, many clinical studies will not have the statistical power to measure differences in kurtosis with much precision, and these may well be omitted.

Looking at the "big picture," if there is no difference in the variability of the outcomes in T and C, then all of these risk terms are zero, since $\Delta\sigma_H^2 = 0$, and so the higher order terms also equal zero. In this case, $\varepsilon = 1$, so the "risk" terms have evaporated. In this situation, the average outcome μ_B suffices to measure difference in value between the alternative therapies.

Similarly, if the risk-preference terms all equal zero, as assumed in standard CEA, then it is also true that $\varepsilon = 1$. If we assume risk neutrality, CEA and GRACE are equivalent on this issue. In other words, the models nest perfectly: Standard CEA is a special case of GRACE.

We have one more issue to consider: the term $\left[\frac{\mu_H}{\mu_B}\right]$ that multiplies all of the "risk" terms. Recall that μ_H measures the average HRQoL level in the untreated sick state, and μ_B measures the average gain in health due to using the treatment T instead of the comparison C. The ratio $\left[\frac{\mu_H}{\mu_B}\right]$ tells us, for purposes of HTA, that the risk parameter ε will be near 1.0 when the mean gain is large, since a relatively large value of μ_B will diminish the effects of uncertain outcomes. In other words, when the new treatment hits a home run in terms of average gain, the "variability" measures will not change "the story" very much. Conversely, when μ_B is relatively small, the variability terms can loom large. For treatments in which there is very little average difference in outcomes between T and C, the "uncertainty" components can dominate "the story."

Alas, one cannot know in advance whether the variability terms that create ε will lead to situations in which ε differs much (or not) from 1.0. Every HTA must collect the relevant data on T and C to carry out the GRACE analysis. The next section explores this issue in more detail using specific forms for the distributions of treatment outcomes for T and C.

GRAPHICAL PRESENTATION OF HOW ε VARIES WITH μ_B

We have previously emphasized that the importance of stochastic elements of value—captured in the parameter ε—differs depending on the magnitude of the average HRQoL gain, μ_B. In this section, we demonstrate this effect through the use of four-parameter β distribution measures of HRQoL gains from both a new treatment, T, and its comparison therapy, C. To make this exercise interesting, we define a comparison therapy C that has higher variance and less positive skewness than the new treatment, T. This may not be the case in real situations, of course, but it demonstrates how μ_B and ε interact. We then vary a single parameter in the distribution of outcomes for T that systematically shrinks μ_B, and then show how this change makes ε larger and larger.

The four-parameter β distribution serves our purposes well for this demonstration. To discuss this, it is useful to first discuss the two-parameter β distribution and then generalize to the four-parameter version. β distributions are also convenient because the range of "support" (the range from minimum to maximum values) goes from 0 to 1, just as our GRACE model uses HRQoL measures that range from 0 to 1. This will, we hope, demonstrate the utility of this distribution in portraying health outcomes.[8]

The two-parameter β model is defined by α, the location parameter, and β, the shape parameter. The distributional statistics are as follows:

$$\text{Mean} = \mu = \frac{\alpha}{\alpha + \beta} \quad \text{so} \ (1 - \mu) = \frac{\beta}{\alpha + \beta} \tag{3.2a}$$

$$\text{Mode} = \frac{\alpha - 1}{\alpha + \beta - 2} \qquad (3.2b)$$

$$\text{Variance} = \frac{\alpha\beta}{(\alpha+\beta)^2 \sqrt{\alpha+\beta+1}} = \frac{\mu(1-\mu)}{\sqrt{\alpha+\beta+1}} \qquad (3.2c)$$

$$\text{Skewness} = \frac{2(\beta-\alpha)\sqrt{\alpha+\beta+1}}{\left[(\alpha+\beta+2)\sqrt{\alpha\beta}\right]}$$

$$\approx \frac{2(\beta-\alpha)}{\sqrt{\alpha+\beta+2}\sqrt{\alpha\beta}} \quad \text{for "large" values of } \alpha + \beta \qquad (3.2d)$$

The mean is easy to understand as a simple ratio. For any value of α, increasing β shrinks the mean (and vice versa), and for any value of β, increasing α increases the mean (and vice versa).

For any value of μ, the variance decreases as the sum of α and β increases. This tells us that we can preserve the mean and decrease the variance by, for example, doubling both α and β. For example, if $\alpha = 2$ and $\beta = 6$, $\mu = \frac{2}{8} = .25$. If we double those parameters, $\mu = \frac{4}{16} = 0.25$, but the variance shrinks approximately by a factor of $\sqrt{2}$.

Finally, we can see that the skewness is driven by the difference between the two parameters, $(\beta - \alpha)$. This is most obvious for values of α and β that are sufficiently large that $\sqrt{\alpha+\beta+1} \approx \sqrt{\alpha+\beta+2}$, so these two factors cancel out in the formula for skewness. With that simplification, skewness $\approx \frac{2(\beta-\alpha)}{\sqrt{\alpha+\beta+2}\sqrt{\alpha\beta}}$. The denominator terms here basically serve as a scaling factor, and $(\beta - \alpha)$ "tells the story" about the extent of skewness. Obviously, making the denominator smaller (low values of α and β) also increases skewness.[9]

These parameterizations allow us to somewhat independently vary the mean, variance, and skewness of the β distributions, which makes them convenient for our demonstrations. The one real "wrinkle" is that it is difficult to independently vary means and skewness. To make the skewness larger, we must increase β or diminish α, both of which reduce the mean, $\mu = \frac{\alpha}{\alpha + \beta}$. This is where the four-parameter version comes into play.

The four-parameter β (used in our demonstrations) modifies the two-parameter version by shrinking the range of "support" for the distribution and shifting it left to right as we please. For example, we can make the breadth of support equal to half of the [0, 1] interval and then have the range of support become [0.5, 1]. To do this, we employ two new parameters, c = upper bound and a = lower bound. Thus, support for the distribution of outcomes shrinks from [0, 1] to [a, c].

With this change, the mean becomes $(c - a)\,\mu + a$. This shifts the distribution to the right but shrinks its range of support. For example, if $a = 0.5$ and $c = 1.0$, then a value of $\mu = 0.25$ becomes $0.50 + 0.5 \times 0.25 = 0.625$. A value of $\mu = 0.5$ becomes a value of 0.75, halfway between the "boundaries" of a = lower bound and c = upper bound.

The variance also shrinks. Whatever the variance was in the two-parameter model is multiplied by $(c - a)^2$. For example, when $a = 0.5$ and $c = 1$, then the variance becomes one-quarter of what it was in the two-parameter β distribution. Skewness and kurtosis are unaffected because they are normalized by the standard deviation of the distribution. With the four-parameter β model, we can now independently vary means and skewness.

To demonstrate the effect of μ_B on ε, we have created two synthetic medical interventions. The "comparison" intervention, C, has β parameters of $\alpha = 2$, $\beta = 3$, and "shift" parameters of $c = 0.8$, $a = 0$. The unshifted (two-parameter) mean is $\mu_C = \dfrac{2}{5} = 0.4$, but the shift to the range of [0, 0.8] makes the shifted mean equal to 0.32. The variance for the "shifted" C is 0.0256. Figure 3.1 shows the two-parameter general shape for the outcomes of intervention C (which are compressed modestly in our four-parameter example).

The T intervention has β distribution parameters of $c = 0.2$, $a = 0.8$, so it covers a narrower range of outcomes, which (as we intended in this demonstration) shrinks the variance. We set the shape parameter to $\beta = 64$, which also intrinsically reduces the variance below that of our control therapy, C. In our demonstration, we then systematically vary α for "T" so that μ_B shrinks as we reduce α.

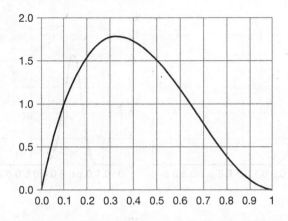

Figure 3.1 The general shape of the "comparison" treatment outcome distribution. In the four-parameter simulation, the range of support is compressed, but the general shape is retained.

Figures 3.2a–3.2d demonstrate the shape of the outcome distribution for T (again, in the two-parameter version). In the four-parameter example, these means are shifted to the right by 0.2 QALYs and the range shrinks from [0, 1] to [0.2, 0.8]. In panels a–d in Figure 3.2, the α parameter grows from 12 to 24 to 36 to 50, with successively increasing means, somewhat smaller variances, and modestly shifting skewness. Figure 3.2a has a slight positive skewness, and Figure 3.2d has a slightly negative skewness.

Shifting the parameters for T increases its mean outcomes. As μ_B rises, ε shrinks. Table 3.1 demonstrates the results. When μ_B is small (near the top of Table 3.1), ε is large, magnifying the difference in mean benefits. Conversely, when mean differences are large (bottom of Table 3.1), ε does not differ meaningfully from 1.0. A difference of 0.20 HRQoL units per year or more (second row from the bottom of Table 3.1) represents a large and clinically significant difference in the mean outcomes of T and C. Conversely, differences of 0.01 to 0.02 HRQoL units per year (rows 2 and 3 of Table 3.1) have very modest clinical significance, and in these cases, the risk profiles importantly alter the effective HRQoL units delivered by each therapeutic option.

The same results occur symmetrically if T has a lower mean value than C, even with its superior risk profile of T that we have created. If T is worse

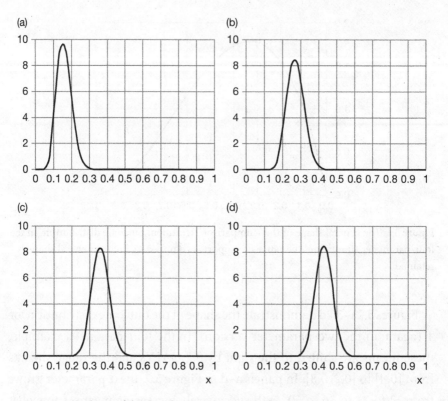

Figure 3.2 The shape of the distribution of outcomes for various versions of treatment T. In each successive panel, the mean treatment benefit increases.

than C by only $\mu_B = -.02667$, then $\varepsilon = -1.84$, and if $\mu_B = .03$ HRQoL units per year, $\varepsilon = 0.75$. The importance of the stochastic elements declines symmetrically as T becomes increasingly worse than C in average benefit.

SEPARATING ε INTO PARTS

As is apparent by looking at Eq. (3.1), ε is additive in all of its parts. This means that we can divide terms such as $\Delta\sigma_H^2$ into two separate variances, one for the T option and one for the C option. Define σ_T^2 as the variance in outcomes for T, and similarly σ_C^2 for the comparison therapy C. Then similarly define $\gamma_1^T\sigma_T^3$ and $\gamma_1^C\sigma_C^3$ as the skewness measures for T and C, and

Table 3.1 VALUES OF ε FOR DIFFERENT VALUES OF μ_B

α				ε
12	64	0.32632	0.00632	2.20
13	64	0.3351	0.0151	1.50
14	64	0.3436	0.0236	1.32
15	64	0.3519	0.0319	1.23
18	64	0.36	0.04	1.19
19	64	0.3831	0.0631	1.12
25	64	0.4	0.32	1.07
32	64	0.46666	0.14666	1.05
50	64	0.5429	0.2228	1.03
100	64	0.6878	0.3678	1.02

[a]As average benefit, μ_B, rises, the importance of stochastic components, summarized in the term ε, diminishes. The β distribution parameters in the first two columns show the exact values used to produce the different values of the average treatment gain, μ_T, and hence the net gain, μ_B.

$\gamma_2^T \sigma_T^4$ and $\gamma_2^C \sigma_C^4$ as the relevant kurtosis terms. Now let us define two new terms:[10]

$$\varepsilon_T \approx \left[\frac{\mu_H}{\mu_B}\right] \left[\begin{array}{c} -\frac{1}{2}r_H^*\left(\frac{1}{\mu_H}\right)^2 \sigma_T^2 + \frac{1}{6}\pi_H^* r_H^*\left(\frac{1}{\mu_H}\right)^3 \gamma_1^T \sigma_T^3 \\ -\frac{1}{24}\tau_H^* \pi_H^* r_H^*\left(\frac{1}{\mu_H}\right)^4 \gamma_2^T \sigma_T^4 \dots \end{array} \right] \quad (3.3a)$$

and

$$\varepsilon_C \approx \left[\frac{\mu_H}{\mu_B}\right] \left[\begin{array}{c} -\frac{1}{2}r_H^*\left(\frac{1}{\mu_H}\right)^2 \sigma_C^2 + \frac{1}{6}\pi_H^* r_H^*\left(\frac{1}{\mu_H}\right)^3 \gamma_1^C \sigma_C^3 \\ -\frac{1}{24}\tau_H^* \pi_H^* r_H^*\left(\frac{1}{\mu_H}\right)^4 \gamma_2^C \sigma_C^4 \dots \end{array} \right] \quad (3.3b)$$

From these, we can readily see that, having broken Eq. (3.1) into parts,

$$\varepsilon = 1 + (\varepsilon_T - \varepsilon_C) \qquad (3.3c)$$

This merely points out that the variance components in ε can be calculated separately for T and C, thus simplifying comparisons of T with multiple alternative versions of C and vice versa.

SUMMARY

Chapter 2 deals with diminishing returns to H. The dislike of uncertainty is a direct manifestation of diminishing returns. With diminishing returns, adding \$10,000 of consumption is not as valuable as the equivalent loss of losing \$10,000 in consumption. The same is true in HRQoL. With diminishing returns, uncertainty in outcome is undesirable.

GRACE reveals a novel "twist" in this analysis for uncertainty in health outcomes of any treatment. Uncertainty (as measured by variance) remains undesirable. Removing that uncertainty creates the value of insurance in health outcomes.

However, because the uncertainty appears in the domain of final health gains, GRACE shows that positive skewness is a desirable effect of uncertainty in treatment outcomes. We call this effect the value of hope. In some situations, the increase in skewness can offset and overcome increased variability, in which case positively skewed variability adds value in addition to average health gains from a treatment.

Our model to assess treatment uncertainty also includes the kurtosis of treatment outcomes, if data exist to measure it. In simple terms, increased kurtosis amplifies the effects of variance and skewness wherever they exist.

As we discuss further in Chapter 9, the data exist in almost every clinical trial to estimate the statistical parameters needed to include these measures of variability in the total assessment of treatments' value. GRACE simply adds the necessity of reporting these data from such studies and using the resulting statistical information to estimate the correction factor ε that is used to adjust average treatment gains that form the basis for measuring "value" in standard CEA.

The Total Value of Medical Interventions and the Trade-Off Between Quality of Life and Life Expectancy

In the end, it's not the years in your life that count, it's the life in your years.

—ABRAHAM LINCOLN

THE TOTAL VALUE OF A MEDICAL INTERVENTION

At this point, we can now summarize the total value of a medical intervention (TVMI). In Chapters 2 and 3, we generalized the willingness to pay (WTP) measure for health gains and showed how to adjust treatment effects for uncertain treatment outcomes. To complete the TVMI, we need two new measures—the improvement in survival probability associated with the new treatment and a way to convert such extensions in life expectancy (LE) into HRQoL units so that we can add them together with gains to HRQoL. Define μ_p as the average improvement in survival probability from one period to the next, and δ as the "exchange rate" between HRQoL and LE. Formally, this "exchange rate" is known as the marginal

Valuing Health. Charles E. Phelps and Darius N. Lakdawalla, Oxford University Press. © Oxford University Press 2024.
DOI: 10.1093/oso/9780197686287.003.0004

rate of substitution (MRS), specifically written as $\dfrac{d\text{HRQoL}}{d\text{LE}}$. Its inverse, $\dfrac{1}{\delta}$, represents the "WTP" for HRQoL gains, but with payment in terms of foregone LE instead of consumption. Because change in LE reflects a change in probability of survival (a pure number, with no units of measurement), $\dfrac{d\text{HRQoL}}{d\text{LE}}$ has the same units of measurement as H. We discuss how δ is measured and what it means later in this chapter. Here, we simply want to establish why we need such a value. With these two new definitions, we can define TVMI using the generalized risk-adjusted cost-effectiveness (GRACE) model formulation as

$$\text{TVMI}_{\text{GRACE}} = K\omega_H R\phi\{\mu_p\delta + p_1\mu_B\varepsilon\} \qquad (4.1a)$$

The term $\{\mu_p\delta + p_1\mu_B\varepsilon\}$ simply measures the ex post value of the treatment to a sick patient, combining gains in both LE and HRQoL. This ex post value is multiplied by ϕ, the probability of the illness even occurring. Therefore, TVMI reflects the WTP ex ante in period 0 in an insurance plan for access to a treatment in period 1. One can evaluate the ex post value of the treatment for people known to have the disease by setting $\phi = 1$.

For another useful way to think of this, we can convert the LE gain into a percentage gain in survival probability, $\left[\dfrac{\mu_p}{p_1}\right]$, where $0 \le \mu_p \le (1 - p_1)$. This simply states that the gains in LE cannot exceed the potential risk of nonsurvival. This gives us

$$\text{TVMI}_{\text{GRACE}} = K\omega_H Rp_1\phi\left\{\left[\dfrac{\mu_p}{p_1}\right]\delta + \mu_B\varepsilon\right\} \qquad (4.1b)$$

This definition comes from the perspective of an individual in period 0 (the baseline period) considering whether or not to ensure access to a medical intervention for a specific illness in period 1, "the future." The product $\mu_B\varepsilon$ describes the value of the average HRQoL improvement provided by the treatment, with average benefit μ_B adjusted by the "uncertainty factor," ε, which measures the change in value associated with reducing or adding to variability in outcomes (compared with the best alternative treatment available).

In this formulation, the individual survives from period 0 to period 1 with probability p_1 and, upon survival, the person is afflicted with the illness in question with probability ϕ. The product $\mu_p\delta$ measures the HRQoL-equivalent gain in survival probability because δ functions as an "exchange rate" between HRQoL and longevity and converts LE gains (μ_p) into the same units of measurement as gains in HRQoL (μ_B). All these components (inside the curly braces) measure the *quantity* of health benefit provided by the treatment. Therefore, δ has the same units of measurement as H.

The expression outside the curly braces in Eq. (4.1a), $K\omega_H R$, measures the *value* of each risk- and severity-adjusted HRQoL gains. We call this value K_{GRACE}. Thus, the TVMI combines improvements in HRQoL (μ_B, adjusted by the uncertainty factor ε) and the gains in survival probability (μ_p, converted to the same units as μ_B by the exchange rate δ), and then multiplies that total gain by the GRACE WTP measure, $K\omega_H R$. This provides the TVMI.

This raises the immediate questions: What is δ and how do we measure it? The remainder of this chapter addresses these questions.

THE INTUITION ABOUT δ

Begin by looking at some common lifestyle choices that trade off HRQoL and LE. One obvious choice arises in the daily act of eating. Almost universally, eating is pleasurable. Of course, like any other "good," eating has diminishing returns. We get "full" and stop eating. Sometimes we overeat and pay the consequences (indigestion, bloating, etc.). One problem with "eating" is that if we overeat by just a tiny bit each day, we gain weight, which eventually reduces our LE through increased risks of stroke, heart attacks, and other maladies.

It is incredibly easy to gain weight over time. A slice of buttered toast has about 115 calories. So, one slice of toast per day equals approximately 800 calories per week, and therefore approximately 3,500 calories per month. That is exactly what 1 pound of body fat contains—3,500 calories. Our bodies maintain a very fine balance between food intake and caloric need to function—a need that obviously varies with occupation, exercise activities, and the like. The point is that if we eat one slice of buttered bread per day more than our body needs, we gain 12 pounds per year. One teaspoon of sugar has approximately 20 calories, so six cups of coffee or tea with merely one teaspoon of sugar has the same effect. One large chocolate chip cookie has approximately 120 calories. Hmm . . . that sure tastes good. Eating one per day for 1 month adds approximately 3,600 calories, approximately 1 pound of fat, or approximately 12 pounds of fat per year.

Now comes the LE effect. Excess weight increases the risk of dying. A common measure of excess weight is the body mass index (BMI). Before reading any further, go to your web browser and search for "BMI calculator." One of our favorites is from the National Institutes of Health.[1] Compute your own BMI. Now look at Figure 4.1.

The hazard ratio on the vertical axis is the multiplier on the risk of death during the coming year, compared with the risk at optimal BMI, approximately 22–24 in almost all studies of this sort. Being overly thin is also risky, but the far greater risk is excess BMI, particularly for men.

Now the trade-off between LE and HRQoL becomes clear. One slice of buttered bread per day adds 12 pounds per year. Over a decade, that adds 120 pounds. For a person 5 feet 10 inches tall, the lowest risk BMI occurs at approximately 175 pounds. If you add 120 pounds to that (one decade of eating one extra slice of buttered bread), the BMI rises to 42.5, and the risk of dying (the hazard rate) has approximately tripled for men and doubled for women. Similarly, one chocolate chip cookie per day adds 12 pounds per year, the same effect as one slice of buttered bread. For those of us who love chocolate chip cookies, they increase

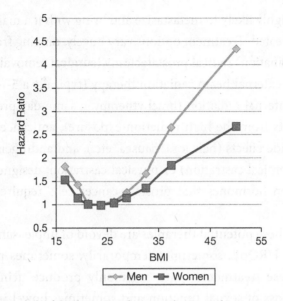

Figure 4.1 Relative risk of death as BMI changes. The vertical axis measures the hazard ratio (the relative risk of death compared to the lowest possible risk for individuals of a given age and BMI).

our HRQoL, but at the cost of lower LE. For a fully rational and fully informed individual, that choice illuminates the trade-off between HRQoL and LE, only in this case, it is not "health-related" QoL but, rather, "gastronomical-related" QoL. Other activities bring pleasure to people that enhances QoL while at the same time increasing mortality risk. Smoking tobacco is an important example, an issue complicated by the addictive nature of nicotine. These are classic trade-offs between QoL and LE.

Let us now turn to assessing LE and HRQoL trade-offs in medical interventions. Many medical interventions—surgical, medical, pharmaceutical, or other—have unpleasant potential side effects. For treatments extending LE, choosing among available therapies (or choosing "no treatment") involves making trade-offs between LE and HRQoL.

In a more specific medical treatment choice context, consider a 50-year-old male patient with advanced prostate cancer, with a Gleason score of 9 or 10, highly likely to metastasize and bring with it a major reduction in LE if untreated. Treatment options vary hugely, ranging from (in single use or combination) radical prostatectomy (surgical removal of the entire prostate) to external beam radiation therapy (typically a 5-week course), high-dose internal radiation (brachytherapy, a same-day procedure with lasting effects from the high radiation exposure), anticancer drugs with numerous side effects (hair loss, nausea, etc.), and androgen deprivation therapy (chemical castration) or physical castration, designed to remove the androgen hormones that prostate cancer cells require in order to reproduce.

None of these potential therapies are devoid of unpleasant side effects that reduce HRQoL, sometimes temporarily, sometimes permanently. Most of these treatments quite commonly produce urinary incontinence and loss of sexual function and sometimes bowel incontinence. Treatments with greater unpleasant side effects can often increase LE by more. The choice among such therapies inevitably involves the trade-off rate between HRQoL and LE. In this case, the choice is most starkly visible when any of these treatments are compared with "doing nothing." For older men with few remaining years of LE, "doing nothing" may well be optimal.

In other disease areas, some trade-offs are relatively minor. Statin drugs reduce cholesterol and improve LE, but many of them create leg cramps, sometimes reducing adherence to the treatment regimen. Other side effects have greater consequence, even if the risk is rare. Every surgery, even those involving cosmetic plastic surgery, creates risks of anesthetic or postoperative infection-based death. The American College of Surgeons has created a surgical risk calculator that takes functional status, medical history, BMI, age, and smoking status, among other variable, into account to determine level of surgical risk. Note that the behavior choices involving BMI and smoking enter this calculation. Again, we have HRQoL versus LE trade-offs. Box 4.1 lists some further trade-offs involving HRQoL and LE.

In summary, "life is full of trade-offs," and the trade-off exists in many ways between LE and HRQoL. In some sense, the trade-off between

Box 4.1

Gain HRQoL with Potential LE or Other HRQoL Losses

Total knee or hip replacements improve HRQoL at risk of deaths from perioperative adverse events.

Lifestyle choices (eating, alcohol use) are enjoyable, but excessive consumption increases mortality risk.

Opioid use reduces chronic pain but increases addiction-related fatality risk (100,000 + in the United States in 2021).[a]

Cosmetic botox treatments improve appearance but can lead to droopy eyelid, crooked smile, or drooling.

Any cosmetic surgery has a small risk of anesthetic death.

Cataract removal has (low) risks of retinal detachment, drooping eyelid, and total loss of vision.

Breast augmentation surgery has low risk of large cell lymphoma cancer, implant failures, and others.

Gain LE with Potential HRQoL Losses

Kidney dialysis extends life at risk of fatigue, cramping, itchy skin, libido loss, anxiety, and the potential triggering of restless legs syndrome.

Cancer therapies (chemotherapy and radiation) extend life with large HRQoL losses during treatment (fatigue, nausea, hair loss, memory impairment, and others).

Open heart surgery with heart/lung bypass extends LE at significant risk of cognitive impairment ("pump head"), sometimes permanent.

Brain tumor surgery creates risks of impaired memory or motor skills or seizures.

Some colorectal cancer surgery extends LE but requires permanent colostomy bag use.

Bariatric surgery improves LE with better weight control with ongoing risks of acid reflux, chronic nausea/vomiting, and food restrictions.

Statins reduce heart attack and stroke risk with accompanying leg cramp risks.

Stopping dangerous addictive behaviors (drug use, excessive alcohol use, smoking tobacco) can create major short-term HRQoL loss (going "cold turkey").

[a]Data from the Centers for Disease Control and Prevention (https://www.cdc.gov/nchs/fastats/drug-overdoses.htm).

LE and HRQoL is just like the trade-off between consumption, C, and health, H, except in this case, the "coin of the realm" is LE, not money.

INTRODUCING DIMINISHING RETURNS TO HRQOL IN THE MRS BETWEEN HRQOL AND LE

Now comes a big puzzle. Standard cost-effectiveness analysis (CEA) states that this trade-off is the same no matter what the baseline HRQoL is of the affected individual. It states that adding 0.1 QALYs of health has the same value for two otherwise-equal persons, one with very low baseline HRQoL and the other with nearly perfect baseline health. The mantra of standard CEA modeling is "a QALY is a QALY . . . ." This emphasizes that the value is the same no matter who receives the benefit or the baseline health status of that person (Williams, 1992). If this were true, then people in those two very different situations should be willing to trade some specific loss in LE for a 0.1 QALY improvement.

This obviously flies in the face of intuition. It is exactly the same issue as the fundamental WTP trade-off between consumption (C) and HRQoL that we discussed in Chapter 2. The only difference here is that the "cost" in this trade-off is not consumption but, rather, LE. Something is obviously wrong with the standard approach to measuring value.

Economists measure the magnitude of these trade-offs using the MRS. In normal economic analysis, this MRS continuously changes as the underlying situation changes.

For example, in Figure 4.2, begin at point A on U1 and increase H to point B on U2. How much LE would the person have to give up to fall back to U1? The answer is that LE must fall from LE1 to LE2 to return the individual to U1, shown as WTP1. Now repeat the exercise beginning at point D on U1, a lower "baseline" HRQoL, and shift H an equal distance to point E on U2. How much would LE have to change to bring the person back to U1? The answer is the vertical distance between F and D, shown as WTP2. This graphical portrait demonstrates why WTP for a fixed health

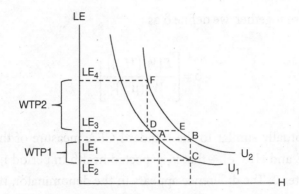

Figure 4.2 Trade-off between HRQoL improvements and LE with diminishing returns to HRQoL. The WTP for gains in H rises as the level of H declines. See text for full description.

gain increases as the beginning health level falls. This is a straightforward result of diminishing marginal utility in H.

THE MATH

The Formal Definition

At this point, we can bring in the formal math to show how this works. Define MRS as

$$\delta = \frac{\text{marginal expected gains from extending LE}}{\text{marginal gains from improving HRQoL}} \qquad (4.2)$$

If we improve LE by a "smidgen," then the gain in expected utility is simply the expected utility enjoyed (measured in units of H) during that extra LE. Define $H_T = (H_{1S} + B)$, where H_{1S} is the untreated illness level and B is the beneficial gain in HRQoL from the treatment. Therefore, the marginal utility of extending LE is the expected utility that the person will enjoy during that improved period of LE, which is simply $E(W(H_T))$. Similarly, if we improve HRQoL, holding LE constant, then the gain is simply the marginal utility of HRQoL—that is, $W'(\mu_H)$.

Putting these together, we define δ as

$$\delta = \left[\frac{E\left(W\left(H_T\right)\right)}{W'\left(\mu_H\right)} \right] \qquad (4.3)$$

It is conceptually similar to the standard CEA measure of the trade-off between LE and HRQoL—that is, expected health in period 1, defined as H_1 in Chapter 2. The difference appears in the denominator, $W'(\mu_H)$, the marginal utility of untreated health. For lower μ_H, $W'(\mu_H)$ is greater, and so δ is smaller. People with lower untreated health will have a higher marginal utility for H and, hence, lower δ. The denominator of δ varies in GRACE but not in CEA. As a result, the "exchange rate" varies with untreated health status in GRACE, but it is uniform in standard CEA. This also means, of course, that $\frac{1}{\delta}$, the inverse, reflects greater willingness to give up LE in exchange for improved HRQoL.

Estimation

As discussed in Chapter 2 regarding the measurement of R and in Chapter 3 regarding the measurement of ε, the adjustment for uncertain treatment outcomes, one can readily estimate δ if an exact form of the utility functions is available (and acceptable) to the analyst. To do this, one simply combines the exact utility function $W(H)$ with the distribution of treated health outcomes. However, some may wish to avoid use of a specific functional form for utility. In this situation, once again, we employ Taylor series expansion methods, which we discuss next.

When avoiding use of exact measures of $W(H)$, Eq. (4.3) is kind of messy because it varies with the expected *utility* of treated health level, individual by individual. The parameter δ is specific to each illness–treatment pair, and it involves the *utility* of health, not the *level* of health. To assess δ

with this approach, individual patients in each treatment protocol would need to respond to studies that measure their individual MRS, and then researchers would average them for policy analysis. This is obviously an onerous burden on researchers and practitioners of health economics and outcomes research.

Fortunately, our old friend Brook Taylor comes to our rescue again. It turns out that we can express δ as a Taylor series expansion involving the usual risk-preference parameters r_H^*, π_H^*,... and measures of *treated illness outcomes* (not the utilities thereof) for sick people and average health outcomes for non-sick people, both of which are readily available from standard clinical trials or general population surveys.

The proof of this has two simple parts, discussed in detail in Appendix 4.1. The first is that $\omega_H R \delta = \rho H_0$, so $\delta = \dfrac{\rho H_0}{[\omega_H R]}$, where ρ is new term that we define momentarily. The terms $\omega_H R$ are obviously part of the standard WTP formula, $K_{\text{GRACE}} = \left[\dfrac{C}{\omega_C}\right][\omega_H R] = K[\omega_H R]$. Since $\delta = \dfrac{\rho H_0}{[\omega_H R]}$, when considering gains in LE, the GRACE adjustment factor $[\omega_H R]$ cancels out. This occurs because, like almost all other applied economists, we use the conventional life cycle model of utility, which implies people are risk neutral with respect to LE. Therefore, we only need to concentrate on the remaining part, ρH_0.

We now define ρ as

$$\rho \equiv \frac{E(W(H_T))}{W(H_0)} \tag{4.4a}$$

which is simply the ratio of expected utility of H in period 1 for an ill person who has been treated to the utility of perfect health, H_0. In general, $0 < \rho \leq 1$, but the "equals" part occurs only when the medical treatment fully cures the disease in question. However, with this definition of ρ, we can use Taylor series expansion techniques fruitfully to its value.

Next, define t^*, the proportional HRQoL loss from treated illness. Formally, $t^* = \dfrac{H_0 - E(H_T)}{H_0}$, where $E(H_T)$ is the average health of treated outcome individuals. For example, if the average treated individual has a health HRQoL score of 0.8, then $t^* = 0.2$, etc.

We can now use Taylor series expansion methods to define ρ:

$$\rho \approx 1 - \omega_H \left[t^* + \frac{1}{2} r_H^* t^{*2} + \frac{1}{6} \pi_H^* r_H^* t^{*3} + \ldots \right]$$

$$\approx 1 - \omega_H t^* \left[1 + \frac{1}{2} r_H^* t^* + \frac{1}{6} \pi_H^* r_H^* t^{*2} + \ldots \right] \qquad (4.4b)$$

Several things are immediately obvious from Eq. (4.4b), which we derive formally in Appendix 4.1. First, if we assume, as in traditional CEA, that people have constant returns to health and are risk-neutral, then $\omega_H = 1$ and all the "risk preference" terms (r_H^* and higher parameters) equal zero. In this case, $\rho = 1 - t^*$. With these standard CEA assumptions, $\rho H_0 = H_0(1 - t^*)$, which is logically equivalent to the term H_1 as used in Garber and Phelps (1997). Similarly, if treatments provide perfect cures, then $t^* = 0$ and $\rho = 1$.

The primary difference between the GRACE value and that of standard CEA is the adjustments involving the risk-preference terms. Risk-adjusted losses are all weighted by ω_H, the rate at which the consumer faces diminishing marginal utility from gains in H. Larger values of the risk parameters decrease the value of ρ. The smaller the value of ω_H (which logically must vary between 0 and 1), the less the treated health level t^* matters, thereby increasing the value of ρ. Diminishing returns occur everywhere! Just as we have diminishing returns in the formulation of K_{GRACE}, we also have diminishing returns to H in assessing the effects of health losses due to illnesses for which treatments are only partially effective.

We now have a way to estimate δ that does not require measuring the utility of the various health outcomes that appear in Eq. (4.3a). That formula is now replaced by Taylor series expansions that only require the "usual" risk-preference parameters (r_H^*, π_H^*, etc.), as well as the elasticity of utility with respect to H, ω_H. In addition, we only require estimates of

t^*, which should be readily available from standard clinical studies such as randomized controlled trials or related studies that measure treatment outcomes in treated and control populations.

Once we take these adjustments into account, we can now restate Eq. (4.1a) as

$$\text{TVMI}_{\text{GRACE}} = K\phi\left\{\mu_p\rho H_0 + \omega_H Rp_1\mu_B\varepsilon\right\} \tag{4.5}$$

The two terms inside the curly braces in Eq. (4.5) are expressed in units of health-related quality of life, H, and K is WTP per unit of health gained, so $\text{TVMI}_{\text{GRACE}}$ is the monetized value of the health gains arising from the medical intervention, expressed as WTP in period 0 in an insurance plan for access to the potential health gains in period 1.

This is the operational definition of the TVMI *before* we account for the effects of permanent disability on WTP for health gains, which we undertake in Chapter 5. This equation provides a way (through ρ) to properly show the trade-off between LE and HRQoL. It reflects diminishing returns to improvements in health-related HRQoL (through $\omega_H R$). It adjusts for the economic value of reducing uncertainty (through ε). Finally, it adjusts for the forward-looking structure of GRACE, showing WTP in period "0" for access to health gains in period "1," once the uncertainty expressed through ϕp_1 is accounted for. If a person has survived into period 1 (so $p_1 = 1$) and has acquired the disease condition (so $\phi = 1$), then Eq. (4.5) allows consideration of treatment values from an ex post standpoint. This formulation also reminds us that GRACE (like other health economics analyses) assumes risk neutrality for changes in LE, so the adjustments using $\omega_H R$ only apply to changes in HRQoL (μ_B).

In a final review of these results, we focus on the effect of permanent disability on the WTP for improvements in HRQoL. Recall that $\dfrac{1}{\delta}$ represents the WTP for improved HRQoL, not in terms of foregone consumption, C, but rather in foregone LE. Define H_{0d} as period 0 health for someone with permanent disability, where $H_{0d} < H_0$. To incorporate permanent disability, define the absolute health loss from disability as $d \equiv H_0 - H_{0d}$, in parallel with the definition of ℓ, the absolute health loss from an untreated acute illness. To incorporate disability, we simply include it in the measure of treated health outcomes, so that the untreated illness level, ℓ incorporates any effects of the disability, d. Just as with health loss from illness, we define $d^* \equiv \dfrac{H_{0d}}{H_0}$ as the relative health loss from disability. Therefore, in the measure of $\delta = \dfrac{E(W(H_{1T}))}{W'(\mu_H)}$, the "exchange rate" δ falls as relative health loss, d^*, rises.

This means that $\dfrac{1}{\delta}$ rises as d^* rises, which in turn means that the WTP for HRQoL gains (in terms of foregone LE) rises as the degree of permanent disability rises. People with lower HRQoL due to disability have greater value from increasing their HRQoL, and hence greater willingness to exchange (or risk) lower LE for gains in HRQoL.

SUMMARY

Traditional CEA assumes that WTP does not change with baseline health status so that the MRS between HRQoL and LE is constant across all levels of H. GRACE generalizes this concept to allow for diminishing returns to HRQoL. This in turn implies that the trade-off rate between HRQoL and LE will differ across different levels of baseline health. People with lower baseline HRQoL should be more willing to trade LE to gain HRQoL improvements than people with higher baseline health. This is particularly important when considering the role of permanent disability in assessing the exchange rate between LE and HRQoL gains.

This discussion, and the introduction of permanent disability in the baseline health state, leads us directly to the topic in Chapter 5—the full inclusion of permanent disability in the GRACE methodology.

The Consequences
of Permanent Disability

There is only one way to look at things until someone shows us
how to look with different eyes.

—PABLO PICASSO

INCORPORATING PERMANENT DISABILITY

In Chapter 2, we discussed how the fundamental valuation of improved
health hinges on the marginal rate of substitution between consumption, C, and better health, H. This trade-off rate is expressed as the
term $K_{\text{GRACE}} = \left[\dfrac{C}{H_0} \right] \left[\dfrac{\omega_H}{\omega_C} \right] R$. We now come to the final change that
the generalized risk-adjusted cost-effectiveness model (GRACE) model
makes. The original model by Garber and Phelps (1997) specified that
$K = \dfrac{C}{\omega_C}$. Technically, this is incomplete. K measures willingness to pay
(WTP) per quality-adjusted life year (QALY), measured in \$/QALY. But
K is simply a measure of dollars, since C is measured in dollars and ω_C
is scale-free. What's missing is the implicit denominator. The complete

Valuing Health. Charles E. Phelps and Darius N. Lakdawalla, Oxford University Press. © Oxford University Press 2024.
DOI: 10.1093/oso/9780197686287.003.0005

measure should be $K = \dfrac{C}{\omega_C}\left[\dfrac{1}{H_0}\right]$, where H_0 is always assumed to equal 1.0 (perfect health) and so is omitted from the formulas. Lakdawalla and Phelps (2020) did the same thing, but explicitly discussed the "phantom" presence of $\left[\dfrac{1}{H_0}\right]$.

Unfortunately, this formulation does not allow for the presence of a permanent disability in a "representative individual." To correct this, we must allow other values of H in the denominator that reflects the presence of permanent disability. It immediately becomes obvious that if we write $K = \dfrac{C}{\omega_C}\left[\dfrac{1}{H}\right]$ and if we allow $H < H_0$—that is, a disabled person has less than perfect health related quality of life (HRQoL)—then the value of K *increases* with permanent disability. This is a radical departure from the current cost-effectiveness analysis (CEA) methodology that reduces the value of improving health for disabled people.

To see why this reduction of value for disability occurs, note that the standard model values improvements in life expectancy (LE) weighted by the individual's HRQoL and improvements in HRQoL weighted by the expected LE of the individual. In standard CEA, the total value of a medical intervention (TVMI), where H_B is baselines HRQoL, is

$$\text{TVMI}_{\text{CEA}} = H_B \Delta \text{LE} + \text{LE}_B \Delta H \tag{5.1}$$

For disabled people, $H_B < H_0$, so changes in LE (ΔLE) are discounted. Similarly, if disability reduces LE (as is very common with permanent disability conditions), improvements in health, ΔH, are also discounted by the (possibly) lower LE_B of disabled persons—the disabled individual may have fewer years in which to enjoy the HRQoL improvements.

This is the fundamental mathematical problem with standard CEA: It unambiguously states that improving the health of disabled people is worth less than improving the health of otherwise-comparable nondisabled people. The final step in completing K_{GRACE} incorporates disability in the basic valuation of QALYs gained, and this unambiguously states that improving health for disabled people is worth *more*, not less, than for otherwise-similar nondisabled people.

The proper way to introduce disability in the baseline value is to replace $\frac{1}{H_0}$ in the K_{GRACE} equation. However, it is more complicated than simply inserting the level of health associated with the permanent disability into the denominator, for reasons we explicate shortly. In the next section, we show the proper way to include disability into the K_{GRACE} equation, and then we bring in the effects of disability on the severity multiplier R and the marginal rate of substitution between HRQoL and LE, δ.

GENERALIZING THE GRACE WILLINGNESS TO PAY MEASURE TO INCLUDE DISABILITY

Replacing "Perfect Health" with "Permanent Disability"

To generalize the formula for K_{GRACE} to incorporate baseline permanent disability, instead of requiring "excellent" period 0 health, we now assume that period 0 health is $H_{0d} = H_0(1 - d^*)$, where $0 \le d^* < 1$ is the percentage of HRQoL lost to permanent disability.[1] The earlier Lakdawalla and Phelps (2020) model and traditional CEA study the special case in which $d^* = 0$. In the more general case, we should replace K_{GRACE} with a more general formulation that accommodates the possibility of permanent disability:

$$K^D_{\text{GRACE}} = K\omega_H R\left[\frac{W(H_o)}{W(H_{0d})}\right] \tag{5.2}$$

The adjustment factor is the ratio of utilities, $\left[\dfrac{W(H_o)}{W(H_{0d})}\right]$, because of the way GRACE specifies the marginal value of consumption. Going back to Eq. (2.1b), the trade-off rate between consumption (C) and health (H) is given by $\dfrac{dC}{dH} = \dfrac{U(C)W'(H)}{U'(C)W(H)}$. This is the ratio of the marginal utility of H (in the numerator) to the marginal utility of C (in the denominator). In the formulation that does not include disability, $W(H)$ is evaluated at $W(H_0)$, and this is replaced in the denominator of $\dfrac{dC}{dH}$ with $W(H_{0d})$ to reflect the notion that the marginal utility of consumption incorporates the reduced utility associated with disability. Therefore, we must modify the earlier analysis by multiplying K_{GRACE} by $\dfrac{W(H_0)}{W(H_{0d})}$ to have the proper perspective on the trade-off.

First, note that this new multiplier necessarily exceeds 1.0 if any disability exists. People should be more willing to trade consumption for H when they begin with less H. The key difference between this analysis and the analysis for acute illnesses is that the disability exists in the base period, and it is from that perspective that the trade-off between base period consumption and potential future acute illness must be evaluated.

As discussed in Chapters 2–4 regarding other components of GRACE, if the exact utility function $W(H)$ is known to an acceptable degree by the analyst, they may estimate the disability adjustment factor $\left[\dfrac{W(H_0)}{W(H_{0d})}\right]$ directly, simply by inserting the values of H_o and H_{od} into the utility function, and then taking their ratio.

However, if we do not wish to employ an exact representation of $W(H)$, how can we estimate $\left[\dfrac{W(H_0)}{W(H_{0d})}\right]$, the ratio of utilities of health in the well state to the disabled state? One more time, our increasingly good friend Brook Taylor comes to our rescue. As Lakdawalla and Phelps (2022) prove,

$$\frac{W(H_{0d})}{W(H_0)} = \left[1 - d^*\omega_H\left(1 + \frac{1}{2}r_H^*d^* + \frac{1}{6}r_H^*\pi_H^*(d^*)^2 + \dots\right)\right] \qquad (5.3a)$$

To simplify this, define

$$\psi \equiv \omega_H \left(1 + \frac{1}{2} r_H^* d^* + \frac{1}{6} r_H^* \pi_H^* (d^*)^2 + \ldots \right) \tag{5.3b}$$

Now $\dfrac{W(H_{0d})}{W(H_0)} = 1 - \psi d^*$. This is the inverse of the term in K^D_{GRACE}, so the multiplier becomes $\dfrac{1}{(1 - \psi d^*)}$. We summarize the disability multiplier as $D = \dfrac{1}{(1 - \psi d^*)}$. With this, the full K^D_{GRACE} expression becomes

$$K^D_{\text{GRACE}} = DK\omega_H R = DK_{\text{GRACE}} \tag{5.4}$$

Looking back over previous "versions" of WTP, if $d^* = 0$, then $K^D_{\text{GRACE}} = K_{\text{GRACE}} = K\omega_H R$. Next, if there is no risk aversion or diminishing returns to H, $r_H^* = 0$, $R = 1$, $\omega_H = 1$, so therefore, $K^D_{\text{GRACE}} = K_{\text{GRACE}} = K$, the original Garber and Phelps' (1997) formulation. This is our final adjustment to the original value of K. K^D_{GRACE} now incorporates diminishing returns to H (via ω_H), severity of illness adjustment (via R), and, finally, permanent disability in the baseline health state, through the disability multiplier D, all of which appear in Eq. (5.4).

Several noteworthy things appear in the estimate of ψ (Eq. 5.3b). First, if people are risk neutral and have no diminishing returns to H, then $\psi = 1$ because in this situation, $\omega_H = 1$ and all of the risk-preference parameters equal zero. In this case, the WTP adjustment is simply $\dfrac{1}{1 - d^*}$. This is what intuition would lead us to in the absence of diminishing returns to H.

Second, all of the effects of d^* are modified by the key parameter ω_H. The faster the marginal utility of health declines (low ω_H), the less the disability effect matters in K_{GRACE}. Diminishing returns to H affect *everything*, including how people value the effects of permanent disabilities.[2] This is why the adjustment factor is not $\dfrac{1}{1 - d^*}$ but, rather, $\dfrac{1}{1 - \psi d^*}$, which equals $\dfrac{1}{1-d^*}$ only when there are no diminishing returns to health and no risk aversion in health.

Third, we can see that ψ depends on ω_H and the relative risk parameters, $r_H^*, \pi^* \tau^*$, etc., all of which are already required by GRACE analyses. This is good news: It means that the analysis to incorporate disability properly in K_{GRACE} does not require any new information except the degree of permanent disability, d^*.

How Disability Affects the Severity Adjustment R

A separate effect emerges with measuring K_{GRACE}^D for persons with disability: Greater levels of disability increase the overall illness severity when calculating the severity-adjustment parameter R, and therefore R is greater for disabled people than for nondisabled people with the same severity of acute illness.

There are two commonly used ways to combine acute illness and permanent disability. One way is additive. With this approach, the net health status used in calculating R is simply $H_0(1-\ell^*-d^*)$, where ℓ^* measures the relative health loss from the acute illness, and d^* measures the relative health loss from permanent disability. One disquieting feature of this approach is that net health can become negative, which complicates the entire model seriously.

One solution to that is to use a multiplicative model, where the net health state for a person with both acute illness and permanent disability is $H_0(1-\ell^*)(1-d^*)$, which is always positive. This has the specific effect of stating that a disability reduces a person's HRQoL less in the sick state than in the healthy state, since $(1-\ell^*)(1-d^*) < (1-d^*)$. We return to this issue shortly because it affects conclusions that we can draw about the effect of disability on the value of improving LE.

Both of the common methods "work" when computing R in the GRACE framework, but we soon discuss a situation in which using the multiplicative model clarifies the effect of disability on extending the value of life within the GRACE framework.

One additional issue remains, namely the distinctions between ex ante and ex post assessment of health loss from disability. An extensive litera- ture suggests that when people become disabled, they adjust to their new situations so that the loss of HRQoL due to the disability declines with adap- tation.[3] The extent to which this occurs does not affect how GRACE works but, rather, simply affects the final value of d^* chosen to use in GRACE formulas.

REDEFINING THE TOTAL VALUE OF A MEDICAL INTERVENTION

Combining the Elements of TVMI to Include Disability

Adding the effects of permanent disability into the value of K_{GRACE}, we can redefine the total value of a medical intervention to include the disability adjustment factor D:

$$\text{TVMI}^{D}_{\text{GRACE}} = K\omega_{H} RD\phi\{\mu_{p}\delta + p_{1}\mu_{B}\varepsilon\} \tag{5.5}$$

Notice, importantly, that the new adjustment factor D applies identically to increases in both HRQoL and LE.

As a refresher, in this formulation, the "viewpoint" is that of representa- tive people in the base period (period 0), stating their WTP for treatment of a potential illness in period 1. Herein, ϕ is the probability of getting sick in period 1, and p_1 is the probability of surviving from period 0 to period 1. Furthermore, μ_B is the average treatment effect in improving HRQoL, μ_p is the improvement provided by the medical intervention in improving survival probability, and ε adjusts the QALY gain by the uncertainty of treatment outcomes (see Chapter 3). Once again, we note that an ex post estimate of the value of treating a person known to have the illness can be attained by setting both ϕ and p_1 to values of 1.0.

The HRQoL Versus LE Trade-Off When Disability Is Included

We began by noting that GRACE fundamentally rests on the trade-off between C and H, the MRS, $\left[\dfrac{C}{H}\right]\left[\dfrac{\omega_H}{\omega_C}\right]R$. Equation (5.5) contains another equally important trade-off rate, the MRS between HRQoL and LE. People commonly must think about such trade-offs, for example, when choosing among different cancer treatment options that offer different combinations of survival improvement and adverse side effects. In Chapter 4, we defined this MRS as δ.

Now comes the complicated part about dealing with permanent disability. Whereas D unambiguously increases WTP for disabled people, and R similarly increases WTP for disabled people, δ has the opposite effect. First, as discussed in Chapter 4, when we look at the modified value for $\delta = \dfrac{\rho H_0}{\omega_H R}$, we see that some of the primary parameters of K_{GRACE}, namely $\omega_H R$, cancel out when valuing increases of survival probability, μ_p.

This leaves us to consider ρH_0, and as we demonstrated in Chapter 4, ρ declines as disability severity increases, since $E(W(H_{1T}))$ becomes increasingly smaller as disability increases. Therefore, the net effect of permanent disability on the value of life-extending interventions is ambiguous. The net consequence depends on the product of $D\rho$. The math gets complicated (see Appendix 5.2), but the basic concept is less difficult to understand. In the context of evaluating ρ as disability changes, greater disability *increases* the value of LE improvements if it reduces "sick state" HRQoL by less than it reduces "healthy state" HRQoL.

The resulting final expression for TVMI then incorporates all of these issues:

$$\text{TVMI}_{\text{GRACE}}^{D} = KD\phi\left\{\mu_p \rho H_0 + \omega_H Rp_1\mu_B\varepsilon\right\} \qquad (5.6)$$

Equation (5.6) represents the final expression to measure the value of a medical intervention. In addition to incorporating a measurable trade-off between LE and HRQoL (through ρ) and the effects of diminishing returns to HRQoL (through $\omega_H R$), this expression for $\text{TVMI}^D_{\text{GRACE}}$ also shows the effect of permanent disability (through D). This completes our final analysis of the proper way to measure value for a person who has diminishing marginal utility for HRQoL and hence also shows risk aversion over uncertainty of treatment outcomes (as expressed through ε).

SUMMARY

One of the most contentious issues regarding standard CEA is the clear implication that improving the HRQoL or LE of disabled people is worth less than doing so for otherwise-similar nondisabled people. In the United States, the Affordable Care Act forbids use of any cost-effectiveness model that "reduces the value of a life because of disability" for making decisions in Medicare or for recommending treatments through the Patient Centered and Outcomes Research Institute. This independent agency conducts "comparative effectiveness" studies of treatments because it cannot use standard CEA models to compute incremental cost-effectiveness ratios.

Attempts to paper this problem over by assuming in CEA that people are really not disabled (Nord et al., 1999; Basu et al., 2020) approach the problem from what we believe is the wrong direction. The real issue is how to properly value medical interventions with and without disability.

The GRACE method directly addresses this issue. Recall that GRACE models the value placed on improving HRQoL and extending LE using the framework of a rational, risk-averse "representative individual." GRACE shows that such persons alter their valuation of medical interventions when afflicted by a permanent disability in three distinct ways.

First, GRACE values improvements in HRQoL more, specifically according to the ratio $D = \dfrac{1}{(1 - \psi d^*)}$, where d^* is the proportional loss in QoL created by disability. The ratio D necessarily exceeds 1 when $d^* > 0$. The extent to which this occurs is modified by the parameter ψ, which in turn depends on measures of the rate at which utility of health declines as H increases,

ω_H, and also through measures of risk aversion, r^*, π^*, and higher order parameters. Just as in all other facets of value, the effect of permanent disability depends in part on the extent of diminishing returns.

Second, in GRACE, the severity of illness multiplier R climbs directly with disability, ensuring that for any degree of acute illness severity, ℓ^*, R has greater value when $d^* > 0$ than when $d^* = 0$ (i.e., no disability). This feature of GRACE magnifies the effects of disability when measuring the value of improving HRQoL.

These changes *unambiguously* show that when the analysis properly accounts for diminishing marginal utility of health, the value of improving HRQoL for disabled people exceeds that for otherwise-identical nondisabled people. Instead of lowering the apparent value in such cases, it increases it.

Third, the situation for extending LE is more complex because (as our analysis shows unambiguously) when people have differing levels of HRQoL, their marginal rate of substitution of HRQoL for LE differs. The "trade-off rate" changes with HRQoL. In particular, GRACE states that people with lower HRQoL should be more willing to trade LE to improve their HRQoL than those with higher HRQoL.

This same trade-off rate affects the total value of a medical innovation, $\text{TVMI}^D_{\text{GRACE}}$, because the same term δ converts gains in LE into "equivalent" gains in HRQoL. This means that with regard to gains in LE, GRACE, similar to standard CEA, can apparently reduce the value of extending the LE for persons with disabilities.

GRACE modifies this result in several complex ways. We have been able to show (at this point) that several situations exist in which the GRACE value of improving LE for disabled people is unambiguously the same or higher than that for otherwise-similar nondisabled people. These are not "weird" situations but, rather, could be expected in general; however, we cannot know for sure until we have better measures of ω_H and the relative risk aversion parameters used by GRACE to calculate ψ and ρ, both of which enter the final valuation measure.

One situation in which we can ensure higher valuation for disabled people is if utility in health has constant relative risk aversion (CRRA).

As we have noted previously, a consensus has emerged that utility in consumption is approximately CRRA, but this leaves no assurances about the parallel parameter in HRQoL.

A second situation exists in which we can ensure that GRACE places higher value on improving LE for disabled people than for comparable nondisabled people. This comes from the choice among methods to combine acute illness and disability to reach a final measure of health status.

For relative losses in HRQoL of d^* for disability and ℓ^* for acute illness, a number of ways exist in the CEA literature to combine them. The two most common are "additive" and "multiplicative." The additive model, where health is measured as $H_0(1 - d^* - \ell^*)$, assumes the effects of the disability and acute are additive and independent. This approach has the unfortunate consequence that it can create negative values of health, whereas most measures of HRQoL range from 0 to 1. This complication has not been fully resolved in the CEA literature.

The primary alternative, the multiplicative approach, states that final health is measured by $H_0(1 - d^*)(1 - \ell^*)$, which must fall in the range between 0 and 1 because both d^* and ℓ^* are constructed so that they must lie in the $(0, 1)$ range. Whenever disability and acute illness are combined in this way, GRACE measures the value of LE improvements for disabled persons as greater than for otherwise-similar nondisabled persons, in addition to the unambiguous increase in measured HRQoL for disabled people.

This occurs because the HRQoL loss from disability in the sick state is smaller than the HRQoL loss in the well state, since $(1 - \ell^*)(1 - d^*) < (1 - d^*)$. In this situation, we have proven (see Appendix 5.2) that increased disability unambiguously increases the value of improved LE. We have not yet, however, found any determinant results when the additive method for combining disability and acute illness is used, so at this point, this situation remains as an empirical question about GRACE showing lower value for treating disabled persons compared with otherwise-similar nondisabled persons.

Of course, these discussions reflect a perhaps rare situation in which the only gains from treating a person with disability come through gains in LE. Real-world treatments that generally improve LE also improve

HRQoL. In these cases, the LE gains have a smaller relative effect on the total $\text{TVMI}^D_{\text{GRACE}}$ value, and the risks that the GRACE model calculates a lower value of treatment for people with disabilities declines. At the other extreme, of course, when treatments provide only HRQoL gains, GRACE unambiguously demonstrates greater value for treating disabled people than for otherwise-similar nondisabled people.

Finally, we have been able to prove that when the treatment does not involve any acute illness, but instead improves LE and/or HRQoL, GRACE shows that the value of reducing the disability is unambiguously greater than for similar health gains to non-disabled people. This occurs because in this case, $D\rho$ cannot be less than 1. This applies both to medical treatments and accommodative devices and even to improvements in buildings and surrounding areas as required by the Americans with Disabilities Act. We develop this finding more formally in Chapter 9.

This stands in complete contrast to the traditional CE model, which (as noted above) unambiguously reduces the value of health improvements for disabled persons relative to otherwise-similar nondisabled persons.

Multiperiod Models

> The only reason for time is so that everything doesn't happen at once.
>
> —ATTRIBUTED TO ALBERT EINSTEIN

MOVING FROM SINGLE-PERIOD TO MULTIPERIOD GRACE MODELS

Introduction and Definitions

The original generalized risk-adjusted cost-effectiveness (GRACE) model formulation employed a static two-period setting in which patients are healthy in period 0 and potentially sick in period 1. Nonetheless, this static framework can be expanded to include multiperiod, dynamic treatment contexts and models—for example, Markov models (Lakdawalla and Phelps, 2022).

As we previously discussed in Chapters 2–5 regarding measuring components of GRACE such as R, D, δ and ε, analysts can assume a specific functional form for $W(H)$ with appropriate parameters that allow the full expression of the utility created by various levels of health. The same will hold in this chapter: The Taylor series approximations involved in the component parts of GRACE can be replaced with "exact" measures once an exact utility function is assumed. Although this simplifies the mathematics considerably, some analysts may prefer to avoid making this specific assumption and instead use Taylor series expansion methods as discussed in previous chapters. The remainder of this chapter assumes that the more general Taylor series approach applies. However, Appendix 6.1 details the methods for calculating the value of medical interventions when an exact utility function is used.

Many of the parameters in the $\text{TVMI}^D_{\text{GRACE}}$ measure of value might vary over time. This is assuredly the case, for example, with respect to progressive neurological diseases such as Duchenne muscular dystrophy, amyotrophic lateral sclerosis (also known widely as Lou Gehrig's disease), and Alzheimer's disease. Illness severity would increase over time, making R larger for treatment of acute diseases. With lower HRQoL, people with disabilities would, using GRACE models, have a greater willingness to trade LE for HRQoL gains, and this effect could increase over time with degenerative illnesses. Mean treatment effects might change over time, and so might variances, skewness, and higher order measures of risk and uncertainty. Multiperiod models to value health care gains must accommodate these differences, and they will affect more parameters of the analysis than would be updated in standard cost-effectiveness analysis (CEA), which does not allow for treatment value changing with illness or disability severity.

As complicated as this sounds, we hope to demonstrate that using the multiperiod GRACE method primarily involves additional data analysis to compute period-specific values and to adjust some variables (e.g., R and ρ) as illness severity changes over time. These may involve degradations in health, as with progressive diseases, or they may involve health improvements as new interventions become increasingly effective at reducing the consequences of diseases. An example is the improved HRQoL and LE brought about by such changes as insulin pumps and automatic insulin level detectors for diabetics.

With that prelude, we can launch into the math that is required to estimate multiperiod GRACE models. Begin with the case in which the means, variances, and/or skewness in HRQoL outcomes vary over time. This structure allows an assessment of value over periods $n = 1, 2, \ldots, N$.

The following estimated parameters would then need to be estimated on a period-by-period basis in clinical studies supporting health technology assessment (HTA):

μ_{Bn}: mean HRQoL benefit in period n

$\Delta\sigma^2_{Hn}$: difference in variances of HRQoL benefit in period n

$\Delta\left[\gamma\sigma^3_H\right]_n$: difference in skewness of HRQoL benefit in period n

ℓ^*_n: percentage HRQoL loss from untreated disease in period n

t^*_n: percentage HRQoL loss from treated disease in period n[1]

These differences can be extended to include differences in kurtosis of the outcome distributions if sample sizes in the pertinent clinical studies are sufficiently large.

In addition, a number of derived variables in GRACE depend on treatment outcomes, so they also become indexed. These include ρ, δ, and ε, which would be indexed as ρ_n, δ_n, and ε_n. Furthermore, because R depends on ℓ^*, which might vary over time, it too is indexed as R_n. Finally, because permanent disabilities can increase (with progressive diseases) or decrease (with treatments or accommodation), analysts must account for this evolution when computing ℓ^*_n and t^*_n, the percentage HRQoL loss in the untreated and treated states, respectively.

Now define ΔCost_n as incremental treatment cost incurred in period n, which is equivalent to the incremental reduction in non-health period n consumption, C_n. Where k is the annual discount rate, define $\beta = \left(\dfrac{1}{1+k}\right)$ as the one-period discount factor. We also define $\delta_n \equiv \dfrac{\rho_n H_0}{\omega_H R_n}$, the marginal rate of substitution between LE and HRQoL in period n. Finally, we define p^U_n as the average pretreatment probability of surviving from period 0 to period n, and define p^T_n as the average post-treatment probability of surviving from period 0 to period n. The change in survival probability is defined as $\mu_{pn} = p^T_n - p^U_n$, the average increase in survival probability from period 0 to period n.

The Full Multiperiod Model

With all these definitions, the net monetary benefit (NMB) in the multi-period setting is

$$\text{NMB}_0 = \phi \sum_{n=1}^{N} \beta^n \left\{ \begin{array}{l} [KD\omega_H R_n][\mu_{pn}\delta_n + p_n^U \mu_{Bn}\varepsilon_n] \\ -(p_n^U \Delta\text{Cost}_n + \mu_{pn}\text{Cost}_n^T) \end{array} \right\} \tag{6.1a}$$

where, as a reminder, $KD\omega_H R_n = \dfrac{K\omega_H R_n}{1-\psi d^*} = K_{\text{GRACE}}^D$ for each period. Thus, in this sense, willingness to pay (WTP) can vary period by period because illness severity can vary by period, and hence also R_n. However, d^* and hence D all reflect period 0 decision-making and therefore are not subscripted by n.

We can also write Eq. (6.1a) as

$$\text{NMB}_0 = \phi \sum_{n=1}^{N} \beta^n \left\{ \begin{array}{l} [KD][\mu_{pn}H_0\rho_n + p_n^U \omega_H R_n\mu_{Bn}\varepsilon_n] \\ -[p_n^U \Delta\text{Cost}_n + \mu_{pn}\text{Cost}_n^T] \end{array} \right\} \tag{6.1b}$$

This makes two changes from Eq. (6.1a). First, it makes the substitution using $\delta = \dfrac{H_0\rho}{\omega_H R}$, reflecting the ability to estimate δ using Eqs. (4.4a) and (4.4b), which employ the Taylor series expansion method. Second, this substitution shows us that the adjustment for declining marginal utility of health, ω_H, and the severity ratio R_n apply only to gains in HRQoL, expressed as $\omega_H R_n \mu_{Bn}$. All the health benefits—from both LE gains and HRQoL gains—are valued according to the disability-adjusted WTP measure, KD.

It might seem odd at first to have two components in the expression for cost in Eqs. (6.1a) and (6.1b), but they correspond to two different aspects of cost growth. First, presume that the new treatment, T, has no effect on LE. If this were true, costs might still change if $\Delta\text{Cost}_n \neq 0$. The first component, $p_n^U \Delta\text{Cost}_n$, accounts for this effect by measuring the treatment costs accrued over the baseline "untreated" survival probability, p_n^U. The second term accounts for what happens if LE changes: During the additional life expectancy period, the individual accrues $Cost_n^T$, weighted by the change in life expectancy, μ_{pn}. To see this differently, we can rewrite Eq. (6.1b) as

$$NMB_0 = \phi \sum_{n=1}^{N} \beta^n KD \left\{ \mu_{Pn}(H_0\rho_n - Cost_n^T) + p_n^U(\omega_H R_n \mu_{Bn} \varepsilon_n - \Delta Cost_n) \right\}$$
(6.1c)

This groups together the net benefits associated with LE gains, μ_{Pn}, converted into HRQoL value with $H_0\rho_n$, and those associated with the HRQoL gains that occur without including the LE gains, μ_{Bn}, plus its "modifiers," the latter only occurring with untreated survival probability, p_n^U.

This entire multiperiod model is conceptually the same as the single-period net value, except that each parameter is time-dependent. If we dismantle Eq. (6.1b), we can see that

$$\text{Per period benefit} = KD\left[\mu_{pn}H_0\rho_n + p_n^U \omega_H R_n \mu_{Bn} \varepsilon_n \right] \quad (6.1d)$$

This is the same as the period 1 benefit defined earlier (with K multiplied by D), except that all parameters and values inside the square brackets are now potentially time-dependent.

The remainder of Eq. (6.1b) included the summation terms, $\phi \sum_{n=1}^{N} \beta^n$, which simply add up the values across periods, discounting in the usual fashion. Again, note that because of the term ϕ, the total value of the medical intervention (TVMI) is valued from the perspective of how much a person will pay in period 0 to add access to treatment T to a lifetime insurance policy. This person does not yet know if they will fall sick with the illness that T treats. If valuing from the perspective of somebody known to have the illness or injury in question, simply set $\phi = 1$.

Equations (6.1a) and (6.1b) essentially provide the "bookkeeping" necessary to estimate NMB over time. It is both reasonable and practical to assume that the risk-preference parameters such as ω_H, r_H^* and higher order risk parameters are stationary, so the data collection to carry out the multiperiod analysis would then rest entirely in the domain of clinical and/or modeling studies that estimate means, variances, skewness, etc. of the distributions of treatment outcomes in the treatment and its comparison (or "control"). The untreated illness severity term, ℓ_n^*, and the treated severity outcome, t_n^*, could either rise or fall over time, depending on the profile of treatment effects and the time path of severity for untreated illness.

Commonly, studies measuring the value of medical interventions that extend LE estimate the value $\mu_{pn} = p_n^T - p_n^U$ for each of the relevant n periods. This is commonly estimated, for example, using Kaplan–Meier estimators (Kaplan and Meier, 1958), which show the time paths of LE for treated and untreated subjects and estimate their difference over time. This approach assumes a constant hazard ratio, which is the ratio between the one-period survival rate of the treated group to the one-period survival rate of the control group. It is widely used in clinical studies because it can account for censored data—for example, loss of a patient to follow-up over time.

Decision Rule

A suitable incremental generalized risk-adjusted cost-effectiveness ratio (IGRACER) decision rule that uses net monetary benefits of treatment can be calculated as

$$\frac{\sum_{n=1}^{N} \beta^n \left\{ p_n^U \Delta \text{Cost}_n + \mu_{pn} \text{Cost}_n^T \right\}}{\sum_{n=1}^{N} \left\{ \beta^n \left(\frac{R_n}{R_1} \right) \left[\mu_{pn} \delta_n + p_n^U \mu_{Bn} \varepsilon_n \right] \right\}} \leq \text{DKR}_1 \omega_H \qquad (6.2a)$$

Note that analysts can freely choose any period $j = 1, \ldots, N$ to normalize the WTP threshold on the right-hand side, resulting in this more general expression:

$$\frac{\sum_{n=1}^{N} \beta^n \left\{ p_n^U \Delta \text{Cost}_n + \mu_{pn} \text{Cost}_n^T \right\}}{\sum_{n=1}^{N} \left\{ \beta^n \left(\frac{R_n}{R_j} \right) \left[\mu_{pn} \delta_n + p_n^U \mu_{Bn} \varepsilon_n \right] \right\}} \leq \text{DKR}_j \omega_H \qquad (6.2b)$$

In words, where RASA-WTP represents the risk-adjusted and severity-adjusted version of K^D_{GRACE}, Eqs. (6.2a) and (6.2b) state that

$$\frac{\text{Discounted incremental costs}}{\text{Discounted generalized risk-adjusted QALY gains}} \leq \text{RASA-WTP}$$

(6.2c)

As daunting as this might appear, it is simply bookkeeping to summarize results when relevant parameters in the NMB formula vary across multiple periods.

The Compound Effects of Survival and Discounting

As is obvious by inspecting Eq. (6.1a), the value of future benefits is discounted by two factors that relate multiplicatively: time discounting and survival probability. The one-period discount factor, β, is given by $\beta = \left(\dfrac{1}{1+k} \right)$, where k is the period-specific discount rate. Obviously, β^n grows increasingly smaller as n increases. This is a well-known feature in all economic models involving future benefits and costs, where discounting of future events is ubiquitous.

The second part of future-period valuation, of course, is survival to period n, whether untreated, the p_n^U component, or incorporating LE benefits from treatment, the $\mu_{Pn} = p_n^T - p_n^U$ component. The value of future health gains is reduced by the product of the joint probability of discounting and of survival. In period n, any measured benefits are reduced by the product $\beta^n p_n^U$.

Consider the case in which $\beta^n p_n^U = 0.75$. This could be any combination of the two components. For example, with a 3 percent discount rate and a benefit occurring in the sixth year after treatment, $\beta^n = 0.837$. When the probability of survival for 6 years is $p_n = 0.9$, their product is 0.75 (rounding slightly). This is how much "present-value-and-survival-probability" adjusted benefits are worth in year 6. This product affects every term in the summation of benefits shown in Eqs. (6.1a) and (6.1b).

ANOTHER WAY OF VIEWING THE RESULTS

Some people may find it disquieting to think about WTP as varying from period to period, as Eqs. (6.2a) and (6.2b) highlight. The mathematics here give us another way to think about it. An important property of multiplication is that it is associative. This simply means that $(A \times B) \times C = A \times (B \times C)$.

This allows us to recast the GRACE results so that they are always worth KD in each period. This requires adjusting the amount of "equivalent" quality-adjusted life years (QALYs) produced to become "value-adjusted QALYs" (VA-QALYs). To see this, begin with the per-period benefit measure, but to simplify the discussion, assume that $\phi = 1$ and $p_n^U = 1$ so we are doing an ex post value analysis for a person who has survived into the period and has the disease or injury in question. The value measure in period n is

$$\left[KD\right]\left[\mu_{pn}\rho_n H_0 + \omega_H R_n \mu_{Bn} \varepsilon_n\right] \qquad (6.3)$$

Starting with the gain in LE and taking advantage of the associative property of multiplication, we could write the LE gain as $KD \times \{[\rho_n H_0][\mu_{pn}]\}$. Now, by our new definition, the WTP is always KD per QALY and $\{[\rho_n H_0]\mu_{pn}\}$ is the "value-adjusted" equivalent gain in QALYs by increasing LE.

Similarly, the gain in HRQoL can be broken apart, so that KD remains as the disability-adjusted WTP per QALY and the actual improvement in HRQoL is μ_{Bn}. This gets "value-adjusted" by $\{\omega_H R_n \varepsilon_n\}$. Therefore, the VA-QALY gain through HRQoL improvements is $\{\omega_H R_n \varepsilon_n\}\mu_{Bn}$. Recall that ω_H adjusts for diminishing marginal utility in health; R_n adjusts for severity of illness; and ε_n adjusts for differences in variance, skewness, and other higher order terms, as available, representing the value of insurance (variance), the value of hope (skewness), and so forth. All of these VA-QALYs are valued at the disability-adjusted term KD. If $D = 1$, when no permanent disability is present, K simply represents that traditional WTP value in standard CEA.

This approach sidesteps a distinction made in the original formulation of GRACE—that between the preferences of individuals for health improvements and the physical effects of the treatment in question. This reformulation folds preference effects and treatment effects together into the VA-QALY for purposes of maintaining a constant WTP for a unit of health improvement. Each formulation is mathematically correct and has no effect on the $\text{TVMI}_{\text{GRACE}}$ measures; choosing between them is a matter of preferences, not of logic. Combining the multiplier with the amounts of health produced, μ_{Pn} for LE gains and μ_{Bn} for HRQoL gains, may help some people gain a better understanding of the implications of GRACE.

RECAPITULATION

As complex as this multiperiod formulation looks, it is nearly identical conceptually to the single-period model set forth in previous chapters. For most new HTA studies, the requisite measures of risk preferences $(r_H^*, \pi_h^*, \text{and}\, \tau_H^*)$ will have been measured by specialists in such studies and need not be repeated in each clinical study. Once these parameter estimates are in hand, the data are "there" to fully implement GRACE in standard clinical studies. The only new "requirement" is to report these higher order measures of treatment outcome uncertainty and include them in the analysis.

GRACE treats intertemporal discounting the same way CEA does, so the notation in Eqs. (6.1a) and (6.1b) referring to this is the same, and the expressions involving $\sum_{n=1}^{N} \beta^n$ are analogous to what one would find in traditional CEA. The "summation" parts involve adding up over all pertinent years in analyzing the medical intervention.

The only real issue with multiperiod models is that a number of the component parts may vary with time, so analysts must undertake further research to measure these components in each period.

Thus, we can see that the multiperiod approach to GRACE really differs from standard CEA only in the requirement that clinical study analysts report not only average differences between T and C on a period-by-period basis (as they would currently do) but also variances, skewness, and, if possible, kurtosis of the distributions of outcomes for T and C, all on a period-by-period basis. Then Eqs. (6.1a) and (6.1b) provide the proper structure for what is essentially a complicated bookkeeping operation, albeit one that also requires period-specific parameters. Equations (6.2a) and (6.2b) provide proper decision rules in the same context. Most of these extra analyses would come from data already at hand in clinical studies of treatment effectiveness and, as such, should not create large extra burdens upon those implementing GRACE methods. Increased sample sizes to allow proper estimation of these statistical parameters may be necessary, an issue that we leave for experts in that area, such as in biostatistics.

In Search of Decision Thresholds

> Spending $1 for a brand new house would feel very, very good.
> Spending $1,000 for a ham sandwich would feel very, very
> bad. Spending $19,000 for a small family car would feel, well,
> more or less right. But as with physical pain, fiscal pain can de-
> pend on the individual, and everyone has a different threshold.
>
> —JEFFREY KLUGER

INTRODUCTION

Cost-effectiveness analysis (CEA) is all for naught unless decision-makers have available (and use) a "threshold" willingness to pay (WTP). Treatments with incremental cost-effectiveness ratios (ICERs) lower than the threshold are "good investments" or "efficient" or "of good value." Treatments with ratios above the threshold are undesirably inefficient or "of poor value."

Recall the goal in determining the proper threshold. In the general economic model as set forth by Garber and Phelps (1997), the threshold is the "opportunity cost" of goods and services ("consumption" or "C") given up to expand medical treatment that improves health. But it was not always that way. Before formal justification of CEA, a number of alternative methods emerged to estimate the decision threshold. The most prominent of these were "league tables" and transformations of estimates

Valuing Health. Charles E. Phelps and Darius N. Lakdawalla, Oxford University Press. © Oxford University Press 2024.
DOI: 10.1093/oso/9780197686287.003.0007

of the "value of a statistical life" (VSL) from the economic literature. We next explore those alternatives.

LEAGUE TABLES

League tables suggest whether a medical intervention is "in the same league" as other commonly accepted medical interventions. Alan Maynard (1991), an early proponent of using CEA to determine efficient resource allocation in the British National Health Service (NHS), thought of the problem in terms of the NHS, a centralized nonmarket entity, re-creating the efficiency that competitive markets might produce but bypassing the distributional concerns that competitive markets raise. To Maynard, CEA (based on quality-adjusted life years [QALYs]) could help reproduce market efficiency within a collectivist, single-payer health care system.

Maynard published a table of what he described as "guesstimates" of the incremental cost-effectiveness of a number of interventions. He did not go so far as to state which were "acceptable" or not but, rather, stated that "the implication of these data is that resources should be invested by purchasers in treatments which produce QALYs at low cost" (Maynard, 1991, pp. 1284–1285).

We also note that these data highlight an issue discussed in Chapter 1 regarding how cost-effectiveness changes as the extensive margin expands. In Maynard's table (Table 7.1), for adults aged 49–69 years, the ICER for cholesterol testing and diet was an extremely favorable £220 per QALY. "Unrestricted cholesterol testing and treatment" had a still-favorable ICER of £1,480 per QALY. In stark contrast, extending such testing incrementally for adults aged 25–39 years raised the ICER by a factor of 10 to £14,150. This provides a vivid example of how ICERs can change as the "eligible" population changes—in this case, by way of shifts along the extensive margin.

The ultimate problem with using league tables is that it is entirely arbitrary to determine a meaningful CEA threshold by defining what is

Table 7.1 MAYNARD'S ESTIMATES OF COST PER QALY IN BNHS (£)

Procedure	£
Cholesterol testing and diet (ages 40–69 years)	220
Neurosurgery for head injury	240
Consulting about smoking cessation (GPs)	270
Neurosurgery for cerebral hemorrhage	490
Anti-hypertensive Rx, stroke prevention (ages 45–64 years)	940
Pacemaker implant	1,100
Hip replacement	1,140
Aortic stenosis valve replacement	1,180
Cholesterol testing and treatment (unrestricted age)	1,480
CABG, left-main, severe angina	2,090
Kidney transplant	4,710
Breast cancer screening	5,780
Heart transplantation	7,840
Cholesterol testing and Tx, incremental (ages 25–39 years)	14,150
Home hemodialysis	17,260
CABG, one vessel, moderate angina	18,830
Peritoneal dialysis, ambulatory, for kidney failure	19,870
Hospital hemodialysis	21,970
Erythropoietin with dialysis (assuming 10% lower mortality)	54,380
Neurosurgery, malignant cranial tumors	107,780
Erythropoietin with dialysis (assuming unchanged mortality)	126,290

CABG, coronary artery bypass grafting.

From Maynard (1991).

"reasonable" and what is "unreasonably costly" per QALY within the context of a given list of treatments. At the time of Maynard's publication, per capita gross domestic product (GDP) in the United Kingdom was approximately £11,000, so one can conjecture (if following current ratios of the threshold to per capita GDP) that the implicit cutoff of "reasonable" might well have been somewhere between heart transplantation and cholesterol screening for younger persons, but the choice is arbitrary.[1]

WHICH OPPORTUNITY?

Maynard (1991) was unwilling to specify a way to separate the sheep from the goats. Given current operational rules in the British National Health Service (BNHS; £30,000, approximately 1.0 times per capita GDP in 2020), one would presume that interventions involving erythropoietin would make people "gulp," but when the widely used dialysis for kidney failure has a cost per QALY of approximately twice annual GDP, one wonders how to make a reasoned selection among these as a "reasonable" basis for defining a threshold, based on Maynard's table.

Assessing the WTP threshold in the United Kingdom leads to a discussion about the proper threshold. Welfare economics–based methods would focus on the opportunity cost of consumption necessary to finance the health improvements, but in the United Kingdom, a different approach has emerged, described by its proponents as "extra-welfarist" but focusing instead on the foregone health improvements within a fixed-budget health care system.

Another early and strong proponent of this approach, Alan Williams, a prominent economist in the history of the National Institute for Health and Care Excellence (NICE) review system in the United Kingdom, challenges this £30,000 threshold, stating that its use forces the BNHS to forego use of otherwise more effective ways of improving the population's health. He describes the opportunity cost of foregone health gains as the "shadow price' of health within a fixed-budget system.

In the 2004 Annual Lecture at the United Kingdom's Office of Health Economics, Williams (2004) stated explicitly that "It is widely believed that this 'shadow price' is much lower than the NICE benchmark of £30K." Subsequent work at York University has estimated that the operational "shadow price" is approximately £13,000 per QALY in real-life decisions within the BNHS (Claxton et al., 2015).

Decision-making in the context of a fixed budget differs in an important way from standard economic models in which the opportunity cost of expanded medical care use is foregone consumption of market goods and services (C in our notation), described as "the demand-side opportunity cost" of health care. In the BNHS and similar settings, the constraint is the fixed budget, described as "the supply-side opportunity cost." There, the health produced by foregone treatments is the opportunity cost. It is easiest to understand this budget-constrained optimization in the context of the wider economic concept of constrained optimization, where one input (in this case, "the budget") is artificially constrained, and then decision-makers do the best they can within that constraint (Phelps, 2019b). It preserves the concept of optimization within the fixed budget but (from the standpoint of standard economic value theory) is the wrong choice unless the budget reflects the proper WTP for health, where "consumption" is the opportunity cost. If the budget is set too low, people would be made better off by reducing consumption of other goods and services to gain more health (and vice versa). In general, this approach introduces a "status quo bias" into decision-making and makes it difficult to correct mistakes in the allocation of funds to health care.

VALUE OF A STATISTICAL LIFE

Introduction

A wholly different approach borrows from a separate literature that seeks to estimate the "value of a statistical life" (VSL) and then converts that estimate to the value of a life year. This presents two issues: (1) Can VSL be reliably estimated from available data, and (2) if so, how does one best convert estimates of VSL into the value of a life year?

The U.S. Environmental Protection Agency (EPA) regularly uses VSL measures while evaluating environmental risks and the value of reducing them. Their description of the method offers the following thought experiment:

> Suppose each person in a sample of 100,000 people were asked how much he or she would be willing to pay for a reduction in their individual risk of dying of 1 in 100,000, or 0.001%, over the next year.

Since this reduction in risk would mean that we would expect one fewer death among the sample of 100,000 people over the next year on average, this is sometimes described as "one statistical life saved." Now suppose that the average response to this hypothetical question was $100. Then the total dollar amount that the group would be willing to pay to save one statistical life in a year would be $100 per person × 100,000 people, or $10 million. This is what is meant by the "value of a statistical life."[2]

Note that this is explicitly phrased as a willingness to pay for a reduction of risk. However, the primary literature seeking to estimate the VSL does not use WTP but, rather, assesses the willingness to accept (WTA) risks, and this can differ greatly from WTP. We discuss this difference later.

The most common approach to estimating VSL uses wage differentials for risky occupations such as logging, construction jobs, and, surprisingly to us, garbage collection, delivery driving, and crossing guards, all compared with alternative occupations with lower risk (see Box 7.1).

This statistical approach gathers data on annual earnings in various occupations and links these with annual risk of a job-related fatality. A typical regression model (Kneisner et al., 2004) looks like this:

$$\ln\left(w_{ijk}\right) = \alpha\left(\text{fatality}_{jk}\right) + \beta X_{ijk} + \gamma C + \varepsilon_{ijk} \tag{7.1}$$

where, i indexes the worker, j indexes the industry, and k indexes the occupation. In this model, w_{ijk} is the hourly wage received by worker i in industry j and occupation k, C is consumption, and X_{ijk} represent "control variables" in the regression. These control variables typically include worker's education, race, marital status, and sometimes job characteristics such as the nonfatal injury rate and the generosity of workers' compensation wage replacement (which varies state by state). The variable "fatality$_{jk}$" is the industry- and occupation-specific job-related fatality rate, measured in annual deaths per 100,000 workers. These studies then assume a typical work-year of 2,000 hours, so the VSL = $\alpha \times e^{\ln(w)} \times 100,000 \times 2000$.

Box 7.1

ANNUAL RATES OF OCCUPATIONAL DEATH PER 100,000 WORKERS

Occupation	No. of Deaths per 100,000 Workers
Logging	111
Aircraft pilots and flight engineers	53
Derrick operators, oil, gas, mining	46
Roofers	41
Garbage collectors	37
Ironworkers	29
Delivery drivers	27
Farmers	26
Firefighting supervisors	20
Power linemen	20
Agricultural workers	20
Crossing guards	19
Crane operators	19
Construction helpers	18
Landscape supervisors	18
Highway maintenance workers	18
Cement masons	17
Small engine mechanics	15
Supervisors of mechanics	15
Heavy vehicle mechanics	14
Grounds maintenance workers	14
Police officers	14
Maintenance workers	14
Construction workers	13
Mining machine operators	11

SOURCE: *Industry Safety & Hygiene News* (https://www.ishn.com/articles/112748-top-25-most-dangerous-jobs-in-the-united-states).

Of course, $e^{\ln(w)} = w$, but the logarithmic transformation is a common approach used to better approximate the statistical distribution of the residuals (the ε_{ijk}) in the regression equation. Thus, $\text{VSL} = \alpha \times w \times 200{,}000{,}000$. To provide a specific example, if $\alpha = 0.001$ and $w = \$30$ per hour (approximately the average hourly wage in the United States in 2020), then VSL = \$6 million.

Challenges for Empirical Estimation

The VSL approach presents several significant empirical challenges. First, self-selection makes the estimates too low for the entire population because people differ in attitudes toward risk, and people who are less risk averse will migrate into riskier jobs. Second, people's estimates of the risks in various occupations are almost certainly biased upward, creating upward biases in estimates of VSL. Third, estimates of VSL using wage differentials commonly omit measures of nonfatal hazards that can also increase the wage differential. Finally, and perhaps of greatest importance, is the distinction between WTP and the related but different concept of WTA risks. Whereas the first issue creates a downward bias in VSL estimates for the entire population, the other three act in the opposite direction. There is no immediate presumption to be made about their net effect; this creates uncertainty about how to interpret any given VSL estimate in the literature. We next address these issues sequentially.

SELF-SELECTION
People have differing attitudes toward risk. In standard models of market equilibrium, those with the least concerns about risk would be more willing to accept risky jobs than those with higher aversion to risk, all other things held equal. This means that the wage differential for risky jobs will understate the WTA premium for society as a whole because those who accept the risky jobs are willing to accept a lower compensation premium than those who did not.

The opposite is true when assessing, for example, WTP to reduce mortality risk from studies of the purchase of safety-enhancing equipment such as safer cars, bicycle helmets, smoke detectors in the home, car seats for children, and the like. Those with the greatest concerns about risk will be more likely to acquire these items and willing to pay higher prices for them than those who are less concerned about risk. Thus, WTP studies capture the WTP of those who elect to purchase these items, and this may overstate the population-wide WTP for reduced mortality risk.

BIASED PERCEPTION OF RISKS

Wage regression studies to infer VSL use *actual* job-related fatalities, not *perceived* fatalities by the workers in question. A long literature in the field of behavioral economics shows that people typically overestimate small probabilities, often by substantial amounts.

To simplify the math, suppose that the actual extra risk in a higher risk job is 10 deaths per 100,000 workers per year. Suppose that (through overestimation), workers perceive the extra risk as 30 deaths per 100,000 workers per year. Then they will "demand" extra wage compensation consistent with that higher fatality rate, but researchers will associate that higher demand with a lower "true" probability. The probability estimation bias of a factor of 3X will translate directly into an upward bias in the estimated VSL by a factor of 3X.

To provide a few examples regarding overestimation of small probabilities, Lichtenstein et al. (1978) measured how well people assessed probabilities of rare but lethal events. They found consistent overestimation of the probabilities of the rarest causes of death. Similarly, teens hugely overestimate the chances of death in the near future—18 percent, when the actual probability is 0.04 percent (Fischhoff et al., 2000). Viscusi has on several occasions studied population estimates of people's perceptions of mortality risk from smoking, where the actual probability is approximately 6–13 percent (e.g., Viscusi, 1992). More recently, Viscusi and Hakes (2008) reported on the results of both a national sample of households with a telephone and the subset of those who smoke and a comparable survey in Massachusetts. The overall perceived mortality risk was approximately 50 percent for the entire surveyed population and approximately 44 percent for current smokers, approximately a threefold to eightfold overestimation.

To the extent that this overestimation occurs in the instance of fatal occupational injuries, it will create upward bias in the estimated VSL. As noted by Viscusi and Gayer (2015), "Because people tend to overestimate small probabilities, when these risks are eliminated, they will tend to overestimate the risk reduction that takes place" (p. 990). Of course, this means that this problem necessarily leads to overestimates of VSL using wage differentials for risky occupations as the basis of the studies.

To put this into perspective, in the United States, in 2019, 5,333 workers died from on-the-job injuries out of approximately 125 million workers, for an annual risk of 0.000043 or approximately 4.3 per 100,000, averaging across all industries and occupations. Box 7.1 shows the risks for the 25 occupations with the greatest occupational risk. Even in the industry with the greatest risk (logging, slightly more than 1 per 1,000 workers), these are small probabilities and therefore likely to be overestimated by potential workers in these industries.

These data make it clear that significant uncertainty may surround VSL estimates in the literature based on wage premiums for risky jobs, because the underlying risks are very low and the major proponents of using this approach themselves acknowledge the potential for bias of uncertain size.

OMITTED VARIABLE BIAS
Risky occupations often also create nonfatal risks and other unpleasant working conditions. Studies that assess wage differentials that cannot also measure the rates of nonfatal injuries and other unpleasant working conditions run a risk of omitted variable bias. If the frequency of these nonfatal risks is positively correlated with the rate of fatality risk, then omitting the other variables biases upward the measured premium for fatality risks, other things held equal. The logic of this is simple: Workers require compensation both for fatality risk and these other nonfatal risks, but if the rate of other risks is not measured, then the required compensation

for these nonfatal risks "loads" onto the estimate of the value of fatality risks. In the context of multiple regression analysis, this is a well-known phenomenon known as "omitted variable bias." When the omitted variable (non-mortality risk) has a positive effect on the dependent variable (here, the wage premium), and the omitted variable is positively correlated with the fatality risk, the resulting estimate of the effect of fatality risk on the wage premium will contain an upward bias.[3]

WILLINGNESS TO PAY VERSUS WILLINGNESS TO ACCEPT

Setting aside the estimation issues discussed in the previous sections, a more fundamental problem is that these job/risk estimates do not measure the desired WTP to avoid risk. Instead, they measure the willingness to accept higher risk, which can diverge significantly from WTP. Michael Hanemann (1991) develops a key insight into this issue when studying WTP and WTA in the situation of unique public goods. He states,

> "If there are private goods that are readily substitutable for the public good, there ought to be little difference between an individual's WTP and WTA for a change in the public good. However, if the public good has almost no substitutes (e.g., Yosemite National Park *or, in a different context, your own life* [italics added]) there is no reason why WTP and WTA could not differ vastly: in the limit, WTP could equal the individual's entire (finite) income while WTA could be infinite" (pp. 635–636).

Perhaps the most famous example of WTP in the literature occurs in Shakespeare's *The Tragedy of King Richard the Third*, detailing the fall of the last king in the line of the House of York. Near the end of the play, Richard, dismounted in a field of battle, knows that he will likely die without a new mount. He cries several times, "A horse, a horse! My kingdom for a horse!" This is WTP, and it is evidently constrained by his (finite) wealth. His WTA in this dire situation would almost certainly have required an infinitely large payment. Soon thereafter, at age 32 years, he is slain by his enemy, the Earl of Richmond, who then becomes the first Tudor King of

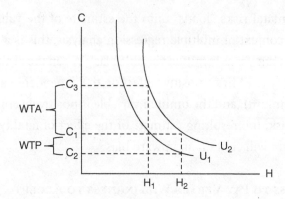

Figure 7.1 The difference between WTP and WTA.

England as Henry VII. In that era, when kings led their troops in battle, being King was often a risky occupation.

Figure 7.1 illustrates this issue in detail. Suppose that an individual begins on indifference curve U_1 with health level H_1 and consumption level C_1. How much would that individual be willing to pay to shift from H_1 to H_2? The answer is straightforward: The individual would remain on the same indifference curve if consumption falls to C_2. The individual's WTP to shift from H_1 to H_2 is $C_1 - C_2$, shown along the vertical axis as "WTP."

Now consider the same person on indifference curve U_2 at the combination of $[H_2, C_1]$. At this point, the individual has the same consumption level C_1 but is healthier. How much compensation (more C) would the individual need to willingly accept a shift back to H_1? To return to the original level of utility (U_2), C would need to rise to C_3. Therefore, the WTA the reduction in health would require compensation of $C_3 - C_1$, labeled as WTA on the vertical axis. Necessarily, because of the curvature of the indifference curves, WTA exceeds WTP.

The real issue for understanding the merits of using WTA estimates to measure WTP values depends on the magnitude of the differences between the two concepts. The answer turns out to be that WTP and WTA can differ by large amounts. Indeed, the WTA can become infinite if the the health space is bounded, as Figure 7.2 shows.[4] Here, if indifference curve U_2 is asymptotically bounded at some value of H greater than H_1 on

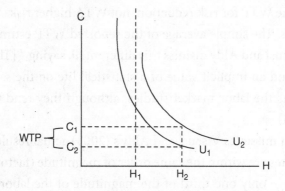

Figure 7.2 Unbounded WTA with asymptotic indifference curve.

the horizontal axis, then the WTA a shift from H_2 to H_1 requires an infinite payment to compensate for the loss of H.

This extreme situation may be unrealistic, but there are several studies that directly compare estimated WTA and WTP values for environmental goods. The first set of estimates highlight the importance of the discrepancy, with an average ratio of more than 7:1 of WTA over WTP (Horowitz and McConnell, 2002). Horowitz and McConnell concluded that "the less the good is like an 'ordinary market good,' the highe r is the ratio. The ratio is highest for non-market goods." Of course, your own health is very much *not* like "an ordinary market good," so the higher end of this 7:1 range may be appropriate.

A more recent synthesis found an average ratio for WTA:WTP of 5:1 for measures involving public interventions that affect health and safety (Tunçel and Hammitt, 2014). We do not know if these ratios would apply directly to WTP for health treatments, but they give considerable pause to the unrestrained and enthusiastic adoption of data from the VSL literature to choose CEA thresholds.

Finally, an extensive review of the VSL literature (Viscusi and Aldy, 2003) provides a summary measure of VSL from U.S. labor force wage differential data of $5.5 to $7.6 million. Viscusi and Aldy also report (their Table 3) a series of studies that reflect true WTP for improved safety—for example, involving higher spending on safer vehicles, purchase of bicycle helmets, smoke detector purchases, and car seats for children. These all represent true WTP for risk reduction, not WTA higher risks in return for higher wages. The simple average of the reported WTP estimates is $2.34 million. Viscusi and Aldy dismiss this differential, saying, "[These] studies in general find an implicit value of a statistical life on the same order of magnitude as the labor market studies, although they tend to be a little lower" (p. 24).

This claim misstates Viscusi and Aldy's (2003) actual results. Although these estimates are within the same order of magnitude (factor of 10), they in fact average only one-third of the magnitude of the labor force WTA estimates, not merely that "they tend to be a little lower." None of the WTP studies in their Table 3 fell within the range of labor market WTA studies ($5.5 to $7.6 million). The differential estimates between their labor force studies and purchases of safety-enhancing goods provide insight into the WTA versus WTP differential. Taken at face value, these estimates suggest a 3X differential between WTP and WTA estimates for the VSL. This does not include the self-selection issue discussed previously, which would imply that these WTP estimates overstate the population average, since those who purchase these safety-improving items may be more risk-averse than those who did not make such purchases.

Using entirely different methods, Martin-Fernandez et al. (2010) directly studied WTA versus WTP in a medical setting regarding various medical interventions. Of the 451 subjects, 404 expressed a higher WTA than WTP, with the average ratio being 3.30. The ratio increased with age and declined with family income. This adds further direct information on the WTA/WTP discrepancy using patients' responses to standard contingent valuation methods.

Spreading VSL into Life Years

The literature on VSL estimates the value of a "statistical life," not the value of a saved life year (VSLY), the requisite value for carrying out CEA. The economic literature on VSL provides some guidance on how to do this. If $U(C,H)$ is period utility, $U_C(C,H)$ is the partial derivative of utility, and

Y is period income, then $\text{VSLY} = \dfrac{U(C,H)}{U_C(C,H)} + (Y - C)$, and VSL is the expected discounted sum of VSLY over the consumer's remaining life cycle (e.g., Murphy and Topel, 2006).

Intuitively, VSLY is the WTP for the utility you enjoy from consuming C and H, plus any leftover income generated in that period that was not consumed (i.e., "net savings"). In the CEA literature, it is customary to simplify this framework by assuming that income and consumption are constant over time and that C = income, so there are no "net savings." In addition, the baseline value of health improvement is typically calculated at H_0. Therefore, the VSLY is constant over the life cycle because it is given by $\dfrac{U(C,H_0)}{U_C(C,H_0)}$, which we define as VSLY henceforth. This constancy of VSLY provides a pathway to converting VSL into VSLY.

With this simplification, one can convert VSL into an estimate of VSLY with specific assumptions about the discount rate and survival rates. To see this, note that

$$\text{VSL} = \sum_{t=0}^{\infty} \beta^t \Pi_t \, \text{VSLY} = \text{VSLY} \sum_{t=0}^{\infty} \beta^t \Pi_t . \tag{7.2}$$

where β is the one-period discount factor, and Π_t is the probability of surviving from time 0 to time t. Therefore, we can estimate $\text{VSLY} = \dfrac{\text{VSL}}{\sum_{t=0}^{\infty} \beta^t \Pi_t}$, in the most general case.

Within the CEA literature, analysts often simplify further by assuming a specific number of remaining life years (N) for the decision-maker and a relevant (real) discount rate. This approach then estimates the value of an annuity of N years at a discount rate of r percent per year, where $\beta = \left(\dfrac{1}{1+r} \right)$, and then divides the estimated VSL by the present value of the annuity of remaining years to obtain the average value per statistical life year (Hirth et al., 2000). Using this approach, which assumes constant VSLY,

Table 7.2 VALUE OF A LIFE-YEAR FOR EACH $1 MILLION VSL

Remaining Years of Life	Discount Rate 0	0.01	0.02	0.03	0.04	0.05
10	100,000	105,582	111,327	117,231	123,291	129,505
20	50,000	55,415	61,157	67,216	73,582	80,243
30	33,333	38,748	44,650	51,019	57,830	65,051
40	25,000	30,456	36,556	43,262	50,523	58,278
50	20,000	25,513	31,823	38,865	46,550	54,777
60	16,667	22,244	28,768	36,133	44,202	52,828
70	14,286	19,933	26,668	34,337	42,745	51,699

a discount rate of 0 leads to a direct measure that VSLY = VSL/(expected remaining life years). Table 7.2 demonstrates this process for remaining life years ranging from 10 to 70 years and for real discount rates of 0–5 percent.

The implied VSLY depends importantly on both the discount rate and the assumed remaining years of life. For any given VSL, the VSLY rises as the discount rate rises, since discounting reduces the sum of undiscounted life years remaining (the denominator of the calculation). For real discount rates from 1 to 5 percent, and for remaining years of life from 30 to 60, the value of a year of life can vary from $22,244 to $65,051 per $1 million of VSL—a factor of 3X. The range extends even further if a discount rate equal to 0 is used (as some argue for in assessing health benefits) and the life expectancy range expands. For discount rates of 0–5 percent and remaining years of life of 20–70, the ratio of VSLY per $1 million in VSL diverges by a factor of 5.6 (comparing $80,243 and $14,286), emphasizing the importance of carefully selecting discount rates and age horizons when using this approach. This gap would expand if Table 7.2 extended to higher discount rates than $r = 0.05$.

Following a common choice in the economics literature, Becker et al. (2005) assume a 3% real discount rate, for which the "multiplier" varies by a factor of approximately 2X between 20 and 70 years of remaining life. The effect of duration declines as the discount rate increases and the actual values (for any remaining years of life) increase as the discount rate increases.

A common way to make a specific choice is to assume some average value of remaining life years for the population involved in the study of VSL. For example, if the average age of that population is assumed to be 40 years, life expectancy tables state that the average remaining life years is approximately 40.

To continue this example, assume that 40 remaining life years is the proper choice. Then at a 3 percent discount rate, the value of a life year is $43,262 per $1 million of estimated VSL. To demonstrate with a specific value, the EPA uses a VSL of $6.3 million, implying that the VSLY is 6.3 × 43,262 = $272,551. This becomes the estimate of WTP for 1 QALY. The effect of the choice of discounting increases as the number chosen as the horizon year increases. For example, if using a 40-year horizon, the ratio of VSLY varies by approximately a factor of 2.33X from discount rates of 0–0.05. At a horizon of 60 years, the same difference in discount rate grows to a 3.6-fold difference in estimates of VSLY.

Dispersion of VSL Estimates

The discussion above provides numerous reasons why it is difficult to estimate VSL reliably. Not surprisingly, the existing empirical literature on VSL produces a wide range of estimates. Hirth et al. (2000) reviewed 42 VSL studies, classifying them by type of model, converting them to a WTP threshold, K, with standardized methods. Median estimates from the different statistical models ranged from $25,000/QALY to $428,000/QALY in 1997—approximately $40,000 to $675,000 in 2020 dollars, a 17-fold range. Hirth et al. conclude that "the value-of-life literature can provide only a rough empirical basis for a decision rule for CEA/CUA [cost-utility assessment]."

More complex models, such as that of Murphy and Topel (2006), calibrated to the EPA VSL of $6.3 million, give a range for a 50-year-old person (in 2000 dollars) from $169,000 to $731,000—equivalent to approximately $250,000 to $1.1 million in 2020 dollars—depending on assumptions about different relevant parameters. A more recent analysis (Cordoba and

Ripoll, 2017, p. 1500) estimates a value of $351,665 per life year for a 50-year-old person, approximately 7X per capita GDP, again calibrated to the wage-premium VSL estimate of $6.3 million for persons aged 25–65 years. Both of these studies rely on the $6.3 million VSL estimate used by the EPA, which (for reasons discussed previously) may well contain significant upward bias.

Summary of VSL Issues

We believe that VSL estimates should be treated with caution because they are fraught with difficulties. The most prominent issue occurs when the underlying VSL estimates rely on WTA values from people agreeing to work in risky occupations for extra wages. The environmental economics literature discussed previously shows that WTA estimates are approximately five times larger than WTP estimates for the same environmental issue. If that 5X factor is applied to the $272,551 value, the WTP per QALY estimate, using standard adjustment methods, drops to approximately $55,000. If we apply the smaller 3X factor derived from WTP/WTA comparison in Viscusi and Aldy (2003), the relevant value becomes approximately $91,000 per life year (all of these are based on the use of a 3 percent discount rate and the assumption of 40 remaining life years for affected individuals). As is evident in Table 7.2, the values also depend significantly on the chosen discount rate and the number of years of remaining life that properly matches the remaining life expectancy of the population involved in the underlying studies.

PUBLICLY ANNOUNCED AND INDIVIDUALLY ELICITED THRESHOLDS

Publicly Announced Thresholds

Not until later in the use of CEA did people start thinking about an actual "threshold" and how to determine its value. Perhaps the most influential of all was a World Health Organization (WHO) publication suggesting that "the" threshold (as a single national value) should be something between 1X and 3X per capita GDP (Tan-Torres et al., 2003). The surrounding discussion concluded that 1X GDP was a very good "deal" and that interventions were still "cost-effective" at 3X per capita GDP, but above that level they were "not cost-effective." Thus, the upper bound (3X per capita GDP in the WHO literature) represents a "hard stop" on the decision rule. Hereafter, when we think about ranges of such numbers, we will continue to think about the upper bound as the absolute boundary between "cost-effective" and "not cost-effective."

A recent WHO study (Cameron et al., 2018) reports publicly announced thresholds that would be used for national WTP-based health technology assessments. Cameron et al.'s data show a remarkable regularity in the relationship between per capita GDP and announced thresholds. Their original analysis focused on demonstrating that these thresholds for the most part fell within the range of WHO's 1X–3X per capita income. A brief statistical analysis shows that the relationship is in fact quite strong.

Figure 7.3 reproduces Cameron et al.'s (2018) original data. These data show a strong relationship between K and per capita GDP, with the obvious anomaly of Belgium ($180,000 per QALY), which has a far greater K value than the "pattern" suggests. The graph also contains the "best fit" regression line, which has an estimated slope of 3.04 (excluding the obvious outlier Belgium). This is remarkably close to the WHO upper-bound threshold of 3X—it simply says that the best fit of these data implies that the thresholds are three times per capita GDP. This simple model explains almost three-fourths of the variance in announced thresholds. This may well be, of course, because these nations were following the 2003 WHO recommendation that an upper bound should be 3X per capita GDP.

It is also useful to compare the logarithms of K and C because this converts the analysis to one of "proportional change" rather than absolute change. Figure 7.3a shows all 17 nations. The obvious outlier here (Brazil) has a very high K for its income level (K = $30,000; per capita GDP = $16,000). The "best fit" regression line in Figure 7.3b omits Brazil. The coefficient is 2.34, which means that for every 1% change in per capita

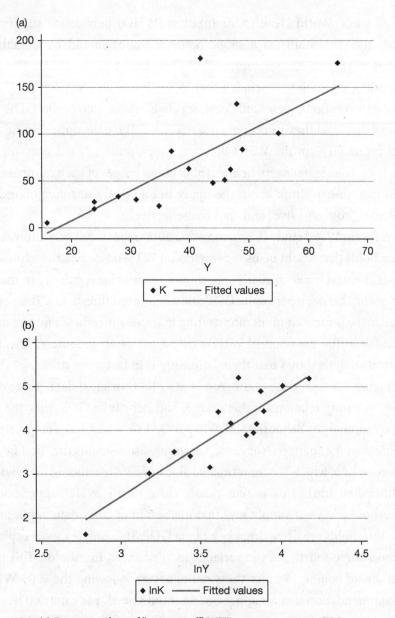

Figure 7.3 (a) Regression line of "announced" WTP versus per capita GDP.
(b) Relationship between announced WTP and per capita GDP in logarithmic
transformation.
Data from Cameron et al. (2018).

GDP, K rises by 2.34 percent. This also means that the ratio $\frac{K}{C}$ rises by 1.34 percent for every 1 percent risk in per capita GDP.

These results call into question the value of having a rule specifying the threshold as a fixed proportion of per capita GDP. The data indicate that for these 17 nations, their announced thresholds, relative per capita GDP, rise steadily with income—indeed, at a more than one-to-one rate.[5] This suggests that as per capita GDP rises over time (with standard economic progress), the relevant threshold should rise, and perhaps even $\frac{K}{C}$ should rise with growing income.

WHO has retreated from the 1X–3X per capita GDP pronouncement, but without offering alternative decision thresholds. Their current stance (paraphrasing) seems to be "it's too complicated to use a single threshold, so don't try" (WHO, 2014).

Individually Elicited Thresholds

Another approach to assessing WTP is simply to "ask people" how much they would value specific health improvements. As one might expect, the results of such approaches might vary considerably depending on the setting, the study population, and, perhaps most important, how the question of value is framed to the respondents.

One Swedish review summarized 383 such estimates (Ryen and Svensson, 2015). The mean value in the study was €97,683 per QALY in 2010, but the range was disturbingly wide—€741 to €892,605—a 1,200X factor. Omitting one large outlier, their mean was €26,189, but the range still spanned a 400X factor.

Ryen and Svensson's (2015) sample included a number of "stated preference" measures using discrete choice experiments or contingent valuation, as well as a number of conversions from VSL to a value/QALY estimate. The authors focused on VSL methods and converted VSL to value/QALY using the same approach as in Hirth et al. (2000), namely to assume a 40-year remaining life expectancy (LE) and a 3 percent real discount rate.

As a reminder, Table 7.2 and surrounding discussion review the sensitivity of results to these two choices.

Ryen and Svensson (2015) found large differences in threshold estimates depending on whether the method used was a direct stated-preference model or VSL estimate with the VSL spread over 40 years using standard approaches. They conclude that if the WTP measure is based on a VSL conversion, it will on average be at least "5.4 times . . . higher than if based on a [stated preference] study" (p. 1297). This bias multiplier is reasonably close to estimates of the same bias as found in studies in the environmental economics literature, as discussed previously.

Ryen and Svensson (2015) also found that WTP seemed to be greater when respondents focused on improved LE rather than HRQoL, with the relative size ranging from 14.0 to 3.5 depending on details of the analysis. They conclude that this difference may arise because the contingent valuations studies regarding LE "may overestimate the monetary value of obtaining smaller quality of life improvements" (p. 1297).

Finally, using a subsample of their library of studies, Ryen and Svensson (2015) analyzed those that explicitly stated the magnitude of QALY gain. They found that the average WTP for a QALY gain is smaller when the QALY gain is larger. This is completely consistent with declining marginal value of QALYs. The discussion about the distinction between marginal and average gains in Chapter 2 (and the differences between Tables 2.1 and 2.2) highlights this issue.

A more recent literature review chose 53 studies that met the researchers' various methodological criteria, separating them into 45 studies with a "direct" approach (asking people about their WTP in some way) and 8 using "indirect" methods relying on estimates of VSL (Gloria et al., 2021). More than half of the indirect method studies were performed in Europe, and the remainder were performed throughout the remainder of the world. Almost all were from high- or upper-middle income countries, and a large majority used contingent valuation methods.

Gloria et al.'s (2021) results (their Table 4) provide a stark contrast to the information captured in Figure 7.3. Calculating the median ratio (and range) of the WTP per QALY threshold relative to per capita GDP, they found that with very few exceptions, the ratio of WTP to per capita GDP was below 1.0. Their summary conclusion states that "our review found that the societal values of health gain or CETs were less than GDP per capita" (p. 1432). The ratios differed systematically. Using their reports for high-income countries, WTP was lowest for "improving HRQoL" (median, 0.48; range, 0.2–24.08), followed by "extending life" (median, 0.57; range, 0.02–10.59), and highest for "saving life" (median, 0.84; range, 0.1–1.41). Not surprising given previous reviews, in the eight studies using indirect VSL methods (and then converting VSL to VSLY), the ratios were approximately an order of magnitude higher (median, 7.87; range, 0.68–116.95).

HEALTH INSURANCE PURCHASES

One study represents a wholly separate approach to estimating WTP thresholds (Vanness et al., 2021). Vanness et al. relied on insurance premium elasticity from a study of Affordable Care Act (ACA) insurance exchange participants in California and Washington and on the estimated effect of health insurance purchase on mortality from a study of state Medicaid expansions. Using these and other parameter estimates, they simulated that 1,869 consumers drop coverage for each $10,000 increase in annual health expenditures, resulting in five deaths and 81 fewer QALYs. This implies a CEA threshold of $K = \$104,000$.

Even setting aside the reliance on a single study of premium elasticity and a single study of mortality effects, this approach obviously assumes that people understand either implicitly or explicitly their increased health risks as they drop their insurance coverage. The probabilities of death and increased morbidity associated with dropping insurance are, as noted, quite small. As noted in the previous discussion of VSL estimates, it is widely understood that people overestimate small probabilities. This implies that they gave up insurance with an overstated assessment of the true health risks and yet still chose to drop their health insurance. If anything, this will lead to an overestimate of K. This approach also ignores the increased financial risk associated with dropping insurance coverage, creating a separate bias.

CALIBRATED ECONOMIC MODELS OF UTILITY MAXIMIZATION

Empirical economists sometimes distinguish between so-called structural and reduced-form empirical approaches. Structural approaches recover underlying preference parameters and use them to make inferences about valuation or other salient aspects of consumer behavior. Reduced-form approaches instead focus on estimating values of interest directly. The drawback of structural estimation is its reliance on specific utility functions. The drawback of reduced-form estimation is its assumption that all underlying preference parameters are uniform and stable within and between studies. Nearly all the empirical literature described above can best be characterized as reduced-form in nature. If reduced-form approaches produce such variable estimates of VSLY, can structural econometrics come to the rescue?

Garber and Phelps (1997) set the stage for this type of work by identifying the optimal cost-effectiveness threshold as $K = \dfrac{U(C)}{U'(C)}\left[\dfrac{1}{H_0}\right]$, where $H_0 = 1$ in the standard practice of CEA. This ratio monetizes utility into "dollars" or other appropriate currency. Phelps (2019a) noted that this also means that $K = \dfrac{C}{\omega_C}$, again with the implicit denominator of $H_0 = 1$. This approach enables all of the studies that we discuss next, all of which estimate ω_C using various approaches. This is particularly of interest because this formulation clearly represents the "opportunity cost of consumption" and because ω_C can be estimated in environments completely distinct from health care.

In recent years, a number of alternative approaches have emerged to assess the relevant utility parameter ω_C and therefore being able to recover the optimal threshold K. We review these studies next.

Value of Extending Life Expectancy

Prominent labor economist Sherwin Rosen (1988) developed an extensive multiperiod model to assess the value of extending LE. His basic concept

Table 7.3 ESTIMATED VALUE OF
K FROM ROSEN'S VALUE OF LIFE
EXPECTANCY ANALYSIS

Discount Rate (%)	ω_c	$\dfrac{K}{C} = \dfrac{1}{\omega_c}$
2	0.81	1.23
4	0.56	1.79
6	0.44	2.27
8	0.36	2.78
10	0.3	3.33
12	0.25	4.00

Summary values from Rosen (1988).

has been embraced by a number of subsequent analyses of the same issue. In one part of his study (his Table 1), he estimates the equivalent to what we have called the elasticity of utility with respect to consumption, ω_c, as defined in Chapter 2. The result hinges somewhat on the economic discount rate, r, as Table 7.3 shows.

Rosen (1988) states a preference for a discount rate of 8 percent (real), a value that is higher than most health economists would currently employ. A more common approach would use a real discount rate of 3 percent, which would place the value of $\dfrac{K}{C}$, the ratio of the WTP threshold to C in the standard CEA model, at approximately 1.5 (using either the mean or the geometric mean between Rosen's 2 and 4 percent values). Rosen's choice of 8 percent places the value of $\dfrac{K}{C}$ at approximately 2.8.

Calibrating Utility Functions Using Risk Aversion Estimates

Two separate studies estimated the key parameter that Rosen did in 1988, but with quite different methodologies than that of Rosen. They sought to identify the optimal value of K and $\dfrac{K}{C}$ by choosing specific functional forms for the utility function $U(C)$ and then calibrating those models using published estimates of the degree of risk aversion in consumption. Once the degree of relative risk aversion in consumption is known, the optimal value of K and $\frac{K}{C}$ can be assessed, conditional on one remaining parameter, and sensitivity analysis across that parameter helps narrow down the relevant range for K and $\frac{K}{C}$.

Phelps (2019a) published the first of these studies using the highly flexible expo-power (EP) utility function (Saha, 1993), a function first explored by Weibull (1951) as a flexible probability distribution function. It includes exponential utility (with constant absolute risk aversion [CARA]) as a special case, and as a key parameter is varied, it spans across a wide range that asymptotically includes constant relative risk aversion (CRRA). The intervening values all include utility that has increasing relative risk aversion (IRRA), which somewhat limits the ability to generalize from this model.

In summary, Phelps (2019a) found that the most likely values of K and $\frac{K}{C}$ rose with income. Figure 7.4a shows the estimated optimal values of K as income grows. The parameter C affects the nature of risk aversion. When $C = 1.0$ (bottom curve in Figure 7.4a), utility exhibits CARA, a concept widely dismissed in the economics literature but shown as a "boundary condition" in EP utility. As C shrinks, utility moves increasingly closer to CRRA utility, all the while having IRRA. At $C = 0.5$, Phelps (2019a) states that utility is "almost CRRA." The shaded area in Figure 7.4a emphasizes the most likely values of C for a range of incomes from \$40,000 to \$60,000, comparable to average per capita GDP in the United States and many European and other highly industrialized nations throughout the world. Within that shaded box, K ranges from a low of approximately \$60,00 to a high of \$175,000, growing nonlinearly with income.

Phelps (2019a) also showed the ratio $\frac{K}{C}$, again plotted versus income, reproduced in Figure 7.4b. Here, it can be seen that $\frac{K}{C}$ rises with income, and again, in the most plausible range of values of the parameter C and

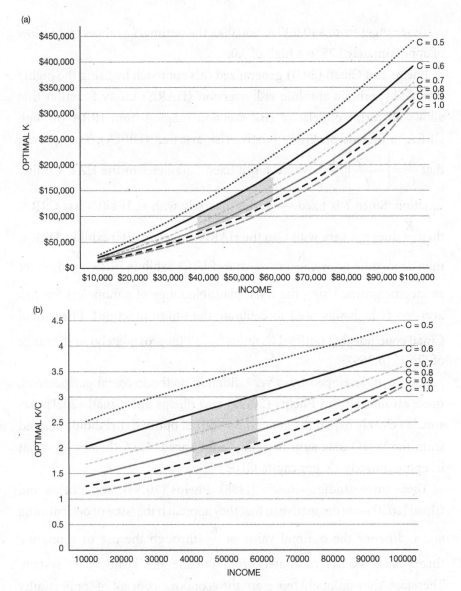

Figure 7.4 (a) Optimal threshold (K) using EP utility function, calibrated using estimates of relative risk aversion. Shaded area represents solutions for incomes from $40,000 to $60,000, spanning the per capita GDP range for the United States and many other developed nations. (b) Optimal K/C. Shaded area represents outcomes for incomes between $40,000 and $60,000, spanning the range of per capita GDP for the United States and many other developed nations.

income ranges from \$40,000 to \$60,000, the optimal $\dfrac{K}{C}$ ranges from a low of approximately 1.75 to a high of 3.0.

Phelps and Cinatl (2021) generalized this approach by using the highly flexible hyperbolic absolute risk aversion (HARA) utility function that allows all forms of relative risk aversion ranging from IRRA through CRRA to include declining relative risk aversion (DRRA). They proved that $\dfrac{K}{C} = \left[\dfrac{1-\gamma}{\gamma}\right]\left[\dfrac{1}{r_c^*}\right]$, where γ is a fixed parameter in the HARA utility function. Since γ is fixed, $\dfrac{K}{C}$ varies inversely with r_c^*. If $U(C)$ has CRRA, then $\dfrac{K}{C}$ does not vary with C in the HARA model. If $U(C)$ exhibits DRRA, then as income grows, $\dfrac{K}{C}$ grows, and if $U(C)$ exhibits IRRA, $\dfrac{K}{C}$ declines as income grows. Using the most plausible range of parameters for risk aversion (which was used to calibrate the utility function), Phelps and Cinatl conclude that optimal $\dfrac{K}{C}$ ratios ". . . sit (approximately) in the range of 1 to 3" (p. 1697).

Although developed from very different methodological perspectives, these estimates from Phelps (2019a) and Phelps and Cinatl (2021) reasonably closely match the general portrait of optimal thresholds derived from the WHO data summarizing "announced" CEA thresholds—that is, approximately 3X per capita GDP.

These three studies—Rosen (1988), Phelps (2019a), and Phelps and Cinatl (2021)—are distinctive in that they approach the issue of determining ω_C, and hence the optimal value of $\dfrac{K}{C}$, through the use of economic theory and models calibrated from outside the health care system. Therefore, they uniquely represent the economic concept of "opportunity cost in consumption" that is central to cost-effectiveness theory.

THE DISTINCTION BETWEEN CONSUMPTION AND INCOME

All of the underlying theory about the generalized risk-adjusted cost-effectiveness model (and indeed, standard CEA before it; e.g., Garber and Phelps, 1997) measures value of health improvements as it relates to forgone consumption, C, where (when income is Y), $C = Y$ – medical spending. Technically, we also need to subtract "net savings," equal to income minus total consumption of all kinds. Currently, the net savings rate hovers at approximately 3% of GDP in the United States—less than $2,000 in absolute terms; as such, it is usually safe to ignore.

Medical spending, however, is another matter because it accounts for nearly 20% of GDP in the United States. Many researchers, and even WHO recommendations (Tan-Torres et al., 2003), treat income and consumption as interchangeable when setting thresholds for cost-effectiveness. When medical care represents 5–10 percent or less of income (or, in the broad sense, per capita GDP), this probably makes little difference, but as medical spending reaches 20 percent of GDP, the difference between Y and C becomes more important.

We can express this issue in two ways. The first reflects back to the initial definition by Garber and Phelps (1997) of the optimal threshold: $K = \dfrac{U(C)}{U'(C)}$. For any given income, Y, as medical spending rises, then C falls so $U'(C)$ rises, making K smaller. At the same time, $U(C)$ falls as C falls, also reducing the optimal threshold, K. Therefore, K necessarily declines as medical spending rises.

Another way to express this is the formulation where $K = \dfrac{C}{\omega_C}$. In the simplest case, when ω_C is constant (and there is reasonable evidence to support the notion that this is approximately true), then K moves directly with C and hence falls directly as medical spending rises. More medical spending increases the "pain" of the foregone consumption (C) and therefore makes K smaller.

Although it may seem implausible in today's environment, nothing intrinsically limits medical spending to 10 percent, 20 percent, or even 30 percent of GDP. As real GDP per capita rises over time (as it normally does), then how fast medical spending grows hinges on the long-term income elasticity of demand for medical care and, in parallel, the rate of innovation in the medical sector. If the income elasticity of medical spending is greater than 1.0 (i.e., health care is a "luxury" good in the aggregate), then the budget share will continue to rise as per capita GDP rises.

A careful literature review on this issue concluded that "aggregate income appears to be the most important factor explaining health expenditure variation between countries" (Gerdtham and Jonsson, 2000, p. 49). This review found that the size of the estimated income elasticity is even higher than unity, which in that case indicates that health care is a "luxury" good.

If this result is generally true, then as per capita GDP grows over time (as it normally does), it will become increasingly important to attend to the difference between income, Y, and the relevant measure, C, to use in determinations of cost-effectiveness thresholds, K. To put this into perspective, the budget share of medical care in the United States between 1960 and 2020 increased from 5.0 percent to 19.7 percent,[6] a compound annual growth rate of 2.3 percent. Real per capita GDP in the United States increased by 1.8 percent per year in the same 60-year period, thereby suggesting that in the United States, the income elasticity exceeds 1.0. Compound growth rates for the medical care budget share of 2.3 percent per year lead to a U.S. budget share for medical care of 30 percent within 18 years and 40 percent within 35 years.

SUMMARY

Where the inference is available, most approaches to estimating K suggest that not only K but also the ratio $\dfrac{K}{C}$ rises with income. This puts into doubt the widely used recommendation that K be some fixed multiplier of C as a general recommendation. Furthermore, as budget shares of health care rise (most notably, in the United States), it becomes increasingly important to attend to the distinction between "nonmedical consumption" and "income" in calculations of threshold values.

These results also make clear that in public programs, a "baseline K," if it applies to all citizens (as does the United Kingdom's recommendation from NICE) will not maximize total welfare of the population unless wealthier people are allowed to supplement their insurance coverage to widen the scope of benefits and extend the intensive and extensive margins of health care use.

In the United Kingdom, approximately 8 percent of the total health spending occurs outside the boundaries of the BNHS, typically with high-end doctors known as "Harley Street" physicians, with yet-unmeasured additional amounts of care sought through "medical tourism" in Europe and elsewhere. Much of this activity, we believe, may be intended to bypass restrictions on scope of benefits and/or extensive or intensive margin limitations of use of medical care within the BNHS.

Canada prohibits supplemental insurance for its Medicare enrollees (a population-wide plan). Nevertheless, many Canadian citizens supplement their Medicare coverage by traveling to nearby medical centers in the United States such as in Boston; New York City; Rochester and Buffalo, New York; Cleveland, Ohio; and Rochester, Minnesota (the "other" Rochester). The extensive travel of Canadians to obtain health care in the United States speaks in part to the higher WTP for advanced health care among higher income people, despite the formal rules to suppress such behavior (bans on supplemental insurance).

Measuring the Risk Parameters

To be uncertain is to be uncomfortable,
but to be certain is to be ridiculous.

—Chinese proverb

INTRODUCTION

The generalized risk-adjusted cost-effectiveness (GRACE) model framework requires new measures of people's attitudes to risk in HRQoL, relative risk aversion (r_H^*), relative prudence in health (π_H^*), and (if possible) relative temperance in health (τ_H^*).[1] Also required are estimates of the closely related concept of ω_H, the elasticity of utility with respect to H. It is also useful to know if any or all of these parameters are constant across all levels of H or if they vary in some systematic way. The simplest assumption is that all of these parameters are constant—that is, constant relative risk aversion (CRRA), constant values for all of the higher order risk-preference parameters, and constant elasticity of utility with respect to health (ω_H). But it is also desirable to be able to assess whether relative risk aversion is constant, decreasing, or increasing over HRQoL—that is, CRRA, decreasing relative risk aversion (DRRA), or increasing relative risk aversion (IRRA). Some important features of GRACE hinge on the question of whether or not these parameters are constant for all values of H, as sensitivity tests in Chapter 11 will demonstrate clearly.

Valuing Health. Charles E. Phelps and Darius N. Lakdawalla, Oxford University Press. © Oxford University Press 2024.
DOI: 10.1093/oso/9780197686287.003.0008

We note here that the concepts of CRRA, IRRA, and DRRA are somewhat unusual in that they really discuss "the elasticity of an elasticity." This is true because, for example, relative risk aversion in C, r_c^*, is really the income elasticity of the marginal utility of income. Similarly, r_H^*, the measure of risk aversion in health, is the "health elasticity of the marginal utility of health." Therefore, when we talk about utility in consumption exhibiting CRRA, we are really saying that the income elasticity of r_c^* is zero, which is equivalent to saying that the income elasticity of the income elasticity of the marginal utility of income is zero. However, if utility has DRRA, then the "income elasticity of r_c^*" is negative, and conversely for IRRA. Although this may sound complex, it is, unfortunately, important in understanding the economics of risk preferences in general and the relationship between r_H^* and ω_H in particular.

The same discussion pertains to the all-important parameter, ω_H, and its "twin," ω_C. Their ratio is embedded in the willingness to pay (WTP) formula for K_{GRACE}. But these are themselves elasticities, measuring the rate that health-related utility, $W(H)$, changes as H changes (and similarly for C).

To begin, it helps to gain a better understanding of how tightly linked ω and r^* really are, whether referring to preferences for risk over consumption income, C, or over HRQoL, H. In the following discussion, we use the subscript C to refer to risk preferences over consumption, but exactly the same relationships hold for risk preferences over health-related HRQoL (H) as well. To see this, begin with the simplest case, where utility is CRRA. Then it is easy to show that

$$\omega_C + r_c^* = 1 \qquad (8.1)$$

Since $0 < \omega_C < 1$ with positive but diminishing marginal utility,[2] this requires also that $r_C^* < 1$. This is fairly restrictive, and in some sense it conflicts with a broad literature regarding the magnitude of r_C^*. In an extensive survey of the financial literature, Meyer and Meyer (2005) concluded that relative risk aversion in wealth " . . . is near, but larger than one, and constant or and increasing slightly" (p. 261).

To understand how r_c^* can be greater than 1.0, we can expand upon Eq. (8.1) a bit. It is also easy to prove (Lakdawalla and Phelps, 2021b, Appendix IV) that where ε^{ω_c} is the elasticity of ω_C with respect to C (there's that "elasticity of an elasticity" concept again!) then

$$\varepsilon^{\omega_c} = 1 - (r_C^* + \omega_C) \qquad (8.2a)$$

which also means, of course, that

$$r_C^* = 1 - \omega_C - \varepsilon^{\omega_c} \qquad (8.2b)$$

If $\varepsilon^{\omega_c} = 0$, then we are back to the situation in which utility is CRRA. But if $\varepsilon^{\omega_c} < 0$—that is, the elasticity of utility (ω_C) falls as C rises—then we can have $r_C^* + \omega_C > 1$. This opens up the possibility of larger values of both r_C^* and ω_C.

The exact same relationships hold for H as for C:

$$\varepsilon^{\omega_H} = 1 - r_H^* - \omega_H \qquad (8.3a)$$

which also means, of course, that

$$r_H^* = 1 - \omega_H - \varepsilon^{\omega_H} \qquad (8.3b)$$

and as before, $r_H^* + \omega_H$ can exceed 1.0, again allowing for larger values of these key parameters. The same is also true in reverse, of course. If $\varepsilon^{\omega_H} > 0$, then that further confines the possible range of values for r_H^* and ω_H.

This brings us to the meat of this chapter. To make GRACE operational, we need to know the key utility function parameters, and it would be very useful to know how they might change as the level of health, H, changes.

We know of at least two methods to estimate these parameters, including "happiness" economics models and discrete choice experiments that ask participants to choose among various pairs of risky choices. However, before we discuss these two methods, we undertake a side excursion into an area of economics that proves to be useful in both approaches to estimating the necessary GRACE-related risk parameters. This side excursion provides details on the hyperbolic absolute risk aversion (HARA) utility function. Among its other benefits is that it provides specific methods to estimate how r_H^* and ω_H change as H changes, which we view as a highly desirable capability. It also provides a direct pathway to estimating higher order risk parameters (as needed for our various Taylor series expansion methods) once we have estimated a few of the basic parameters of the model. We note that GRACE risk parameters can be estimated using utility functions outside the HARA class. For example, a considerable literature has estimated EP utility functions (Saha, 1993) in the context of discrete choice experiments. Analysts are free to choose any class of utility functions. However, HARA has certain pedagogical advantages that we exploit in our presentation here.

THE HYPERBOLIC ABSOLUTE RISK AVERSION UTILITY FUNCTION

Hyperbolic absolute risk aversion utility is both highly flexible in structure and relatively easy to use and understand. For these reasons, it has increasingly gained use in economic analyses when it is desirable to generalize beyond CRRA utility. In the full HARA formulation,

$$W(H) = \left[\frac{1-\gamma}{\gamma}\right]\left[\frac{aH}{1-\gamma}+b\right]^{\gamma} \tag{8.4a}$$

where b can be positive or negative and has the same measurement scale as does H. It is also standard to restrict the ranges of H and the utility parameters so that $\left[\dfrac{aH}{1-\gamma}+b\right] > 0$. It turns out that b determines some key features of what we need to know about $W(H)$, the utility of health, and how it behaves as H changes. The parameter γ is called the "power parameter," and it is closely related to the parameters r_H^* and ω_H that we need in GRACE.

In this most flexible formulation, the scaling parameter a is necessary for full generality, but when we apply this concept to measuring H, where the range is naturally constrained so that $0 \leq H \leq 1$, we can simplify the HARA model without sacrificing generality by assuming that $a = (1 - \gamma)$. With this simplification,

$$W(H) = \left[\frac{1 - \gamma}{\gamma} \right] [H + b]^{\gamma} \qquad (8.4b)$$

This formulation is valid only where $[H + b] > 0$. If $b < 0$, then the utility of sufficiently small values of H cannot be computed.[3]

In this slightly simplified version of HARA utility, relative risk aversion becomes[4]

$$r_H^*(H) = (1 - \gamma) \left[\frac{H}{H + b} \right] \qquad (8.5)$$

When $b = 0$, $r_H^*(H) = (1 - \gamma)$ and the HARA function collapses to CRRA utility. CRRA is a special (and simple) case of HARA. When $b < 0$, utility is DRRA, and when $b > 0$, utility is IRRA.

In HARA, the next higher order risk parameter is relative prudence, measured as $\pi_H^* = (2 - \gamma) \left[\frac{H}{H + b} \right]$, which is obviously very similar to the formula for $r_H^*(H)$ in Eq. (8.5).

Looking at Eqs. (8.4b) and (8.5), is becomes obvious that to use HARA utility effectively, we need to know the value of γ. Phelps and Cinatl (2021) show that γ can be derived from the ratio of $\frac{\pi_H^*}{r_H^*}$. They prove that

$$\gamma = \frac{\pi_H^* - 2r_H^*}{\pi_H^* - r_H^*} \qquad (8.6)$$

This means that if we can estimate both $r_H^*(H)$ and $\pi_H^*(H)$, we have an estimate of γ. Later, we show how to do this specifically using discrete choice experiment (DCE) methods.

In addition, in the HARA structure,

$$\omega_H = \left[\frac{\gamma}{1-\gamma}\right] r_H^* \qquad (8.7a)$$

Equation (8.7a) can be rearranged to show that

$$\gamma = \frac{\omega_H}{\omega_H + r_H^*} \qquad (8.7b)$$

This provides another way to estimate γ using separate estimates of $r_H^*(H)$ and $\omega_H(H)$. Later, we show exactly how to do this using regression analyses in the tradition of "happiness economics." Furthermore, because theory tells us that $0 < \omega_H < 1$ and $r_H^* > 0$, this assures us that $0 < \gamma < 1$.

Figures 8.1 shows the general pattern of what is occurring. If utility is DRRA (see Figure 8.1a), then $r_C^* + \omega_C > 1$, but it converges toward a total of 1.0 as C grows. It is easy to demonstrate in this setting that as C grows, r_H^* approaches $(1-\gamma)$ from above and ω_H approaches γ from above.[5] The same is true when considering utility functions in H.

Everything reverses if utility (either in C or in H) is IRRA, not DRRA (see Figure 8.1b). If utility is IRRA, then $r_C^* + \omega_C < 1$, and as C grows, r_C^* approaches $(1-\gamma)$ from below and ω_C approaches γ from below. The graph of this situation is essentially a mirror image of Figure 8.1a.

As Chapter 11 will demonstrate, the question of whether utility in H is CRRA, DRRA, or IRRA affects the magnitude of important GRACE parameters, specifically $K_{GRACE} = K\omega_H R$. If utility in H is IRRA, values of both ω_H and R will tend to be smaller, so with IRRA, K_{GRACE} can be significantly less than K for many levels of illness severity that help determine R. Conversely, if utility is DRRA, so that $r_H^* + \omega_H > 1$, then K_{GRACE}

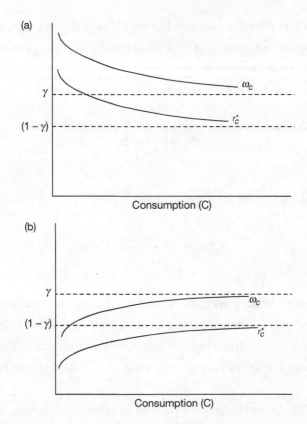

Figure 8.1 (a) Behavior of ω_H and r_H^* when utility of consumption is DRRA. (b) Behavior of ω_H and r_H^* when utility of consumption is IRRA.

can become notably larger than K in many settings because both r_H^* and ω_H can have larger values than if CRRA is the proper shape of the utility function.

By assuming HARA utility, another fortuitous result emerges: The difference between successive risk terms is always a constant, so once we know r_H^* and π_H^*, we know γ, and from all of this, the higher order terms can also be assessed. To see this, begin with the formula for π_H^* and subtract r_H^* from it, giving

$$\Delta = (\pi_H^* - r_H^*) = \left[\frac{2-\gamma}{1-\gamma}\right] r_H^* - r_H^* = \frac{[(2-\gamma)r_H^* - (1-\gamma)r_H^*]}{1-\gamma} = \frac{r_H^*}{1-\gamma} \qquad (8.8a)$$

However, when $a = (1 - \gamma)$, $r_H^* = (1 - \gamma)\left[\dfrac{H}{H+b}\right]$, then

$$\Delta = \left[\frac{H}{H+b}\right] \tag{8.8b}$$

From Eq. (8.8b), we can readily see that when $b = 0$, which implies CRRA utility, then $\Delta = 1$, which is the standard result for CRRA: $\pi^* = r^* + 1$, $\tau^* = \pi^* + 1 = r^* + 2 \dots$ and so forth.

The relationship in Eq. (8.8a) is also true at the next level since

$$\tau_H^* - \pi^* = \left[\frac{3-\gamma}{1-\gamma}\right] r_H^* - \left[\frac{2-\gamma}{1-\gamma}\right] r_H^* = \frac{r_H^*}{1-\gamma} = \Delta \tag{8.8c}$$

Indeed, this repeats itself at every pair of higher order risk terms: The difference between any two higher order terms is always $\Delta = \left[\dfrac{H}{H+b1-\gamma}\right] = \dfrac{r_H^*}{1-\gamma}$, which always equals 1.0 when $b = 0$.

By assuming HARA utility, we are now in the happy position of being able to estimate the Taylor series expansions of every key GRACE parameter and to include as many Taylor series terms as are necessary to reach convergence.[6] Once we know r_H^* and γ, we know Δ. Then, the next-higher risk parameter in the Taylor series is always Δ greater than the previous one. This ensures the ability to reach convergence in the Taylor series expansions for all of the GRACE parameters that involve the risk parameters—R to measure the acute illness severity adjustment, ψ to measure the disability-severity adjustment, ρ to measure the trade-off between LE and HRQoL, and ε to adjust average treatment benefits to account for variability in treatment outcomes.

Another even easier method to find Δ is simply to use direct estimates of r_H^* and ω_H when available, because in HARA utility, $\Delta = r_H^* + \omega_H$. These estimates can come directly from happiness economics estimates by estimating ω_H and then calculating r^* from Eqs. (18.6a) and (18.6b), showing the estimates in the happiness economics discussion that follows. For example, if the estimated value of $\widehat{\omega_H}$ is 0.6 and the calculated value of $\widehat{r_H^*}$ is 0.5, then $\widehat{\Delta} = 1.1$.

As we have noted previously, it is useful for users of GRACE to know whether risk-preference parameters such as ω_H and r_H^* are constant or vary with H. Under HARA, it is easy to demonstrate that for *all* sufficiently differentiable utility functions, the elasticity of r_H^* with respect to H is given by

$$\varepsilon^{r_H} = 1 - (\pi_H^* - r_H^*) \tag{8.9a}$$

To begin, this means that if $(\pi_H^* - r_H^*) = 1$, then $\varepsilon^{r_H} = 0$. That is, if $(\pi_H^* - r_H^*) = 1$, then utility in H is CRRA. If $(\pi_H^* - r_H^*) < 1$, then utility is IRRA (i.e., $\varepsilon^{r_H} > 0$). Similarly, if $(\pi_H^* - r_H^*) > 1$, then utility in health is DRRA. Analysts can readily adjust estimates of r_H^* away from "base" values of H by knowing ε^{r_H} and the percentage change from the base value of H that they wish to make. The difference $(\pi_H^* - r_H^*)$ tells us everything we need to know to adjust baseline values of r_H^* to accommodate other levels of H.

Similarly, for any sufficiently differentiable HARA utility function:

$$\varepsilon^{\omega_H} = 1 - (r^* + \omega_H) \tag{8.9b}$$

Again, the reference case of CRRA is useful. When utility is CRRA, $(r^* + \omega_H) = 1$, so $\varepsilon^{\omega_H} = 0$. CRRA also ensures that ω_H does not vary with H. It is also easy to prove that for HARA utility, $\varepsilon^{r_H} = -\varepsilon^{\omega_H}$.

This relationship also shows why, in HARA utility, $\Delta = r_H^* + \omega_H$. Equation (8.9a) can be rearrange to show that

$$\Delta = (\pi_H^* - r_H^*) = 1 - \varepsilon^{r_H} \tag{8.9c}$$

With negative values of ε^{r_H}, the sum of $r_H^* + \omega_H$ can exceed 1.0. We show in Chapter 9 the importance of this situation.

In summary, within the context of HARA utility, we need to know γ, the HARA power parameter, and then either τ_H^* and ω_H or τ_H^* and π_H^*

to fill out the full array of risk parameters. With this background in the structure and value of HARA utility, we can now turn to the first of two methods for estimating the GRACE parameters that we need.

HAPPINESS ECONOMICS

The study of happiness economics has risen in recent use. The basic idea was pioneered by economist Richard Easterlin (2003). It has blossomed into the "World Happiness Report," an ongoing publication of the United Nations Sustainable Development Solutions Network. This Network primarily uses regular reports from the Gallup World Poll, which is currently edited by leading economists from Canada, England, and the United States.[7] The Gallup World Poll regularly surveys citizens of 160 countries, representing 98 percent of the world's population. Its work rests entirely on self-reported happiness measures.

Necessary Data

Happiness economics begins with the premise that people can report with reasonable reliability how happy they are on a fixed-interval scale, such as 1–10 or 1–100.[8] The methods of elicitation are similar to those used to elicit respondents' views of their own health status, using, for example, a thermometer scale (visual analog scale). For discussion here, presume that the subject has responded to a question such as "On a scale from 0, which is 'as unhappy as you can imagine,' to 100 as 'highest imaginable happiness,' where would you rate your present state of happiness?"

We also envision obtaining a measure of respondents' self-reported health status, typically measured on or transformed into a [0, 1] interval, where "0" is the worst imaginable state of health, and "1" is perfect health— the best that the individual can imagine. Chapter 9 discusses formal methods to obtain such values (see discussion of the Patient Reported

Outcomes Measurement Information System in that chapter), or one could use less complex methods such as a simple thermometer scale to measure health. Our goal here is not to choose among these alternatives but, rather, to discuss the econometric process that follows once the preferred index of health has been estimated.

The third key measure elicited from respondents is a measure of income, preferably income available for consumption after medical costs are removed. If the individual has health insurance, "medical costs" would include both out-of-pocket costs for health care and any health insurance premiums paid by the individual. Again, our goal here is not to recommend the best process to elicit household income but, rather, to discuss the econometric use of the data that would follow.

The Econometric Model

Our next step here refers to a substantial literature in economics describing how to estimate "utility" in a coherent way. For this, we turn to the transcendental logarithmic utility function model, widely described as the "translog" model (Christensen et al., 1975). The translog model provides a second-order Taylor series expansion for *any* sufficiently differentiable utility function. In its basic form, where each x_i is the level of consumption of various economic goods, the translog model is

$$\ln(U) = \alpha_0 + \sum_j \alpha_j \ln(x_j) + \frac{1}{2} \sum_i \sum_j \beta_{ij} \ln(x_i) \ln(x_j) \qquad (8.10)$$

The α_j parameters measure the "main effect" of each $\ln(x_j)$ on $\ln(U)$, the proportional change in utility (U) for each proportional change in goods x_j. Regarding the β_{ij} coefficients, when $i = j$, the β_{ij} terms capture the "quadratic" curvature for each single economic good, and when $i \neq j$, the coefficients capture interaction between the ways any two goods affect utility.

We adapt this approach to study happiness, using the following model:

$$\ln(Happy_i) = \beta_1 \ln(H_i) + \frac{1}{2}\beta_2(\ln(H_i))^2 + \beta_3 \ln(C_i) + \frac{1}{2}\beta_4(\ln(C_i))^2 + \varepsilon_i$$

$$(8.11)$$

This equation omits the interaction terms between consumption and health that the translog function allows so we can focus on the central issues at hand.[9] Real-world estimation can readily include them and, in addition, any other "covariates" that econometricians might wish to include in order to control for other factors that might affect "Happy."

Now comes a beneficial coincidence when using this approach: We can estimate the key GRACE parameter ω_H directly from regression Eq. (8.11). Noting that $\dfrac{\partial \ln(Happy)}{\partial \ln(H)} = \omega_H$, from Eq. (8.11) (and allowing ω_H to vary with H, hence describing it as $\omega_H(H)$):

$$\omega_H(H) = \beta_1 + \beta_2 \ln(H) \qquad (8.12)$$

If $\beta_2 = 0$, then we know that ω_H does not vary with H, so we know that we have CRRA utility. If $\beta_2 < 0$, then we know that utility in H flattens out more rapidly. The reverse holds true if $\beta_2 > 0$. We now have one of the key parameters to use GRACE, ω_H, and we can also determine (importantly) if ω_H varies with H or is constant for all values of H. The "constancy" hinges on the parameter β_2.

Exactly the same process can be followed to determine the other key elasticity of utility in the GRACE framework, the elasticity of utility with respect to C:

$$\omega_C(C) = \beta_3 + \beta_4 \ln(C) \qquad (8.13)$$

We know of no other approach that allows estimation of these two key parameters from the same data set in the same estimation model. Remember that the ratio $\dfrac{\omega_H}{\omega_C}$ is central to calculating the proper value for

K_{GRACE}, so being able to estimate both of these parameters together has potentially significant value.[10]

Turning Happiness Parameters into GRACE Parameters

Having completed the key task of estimating ω_H and understanding how it might vary with H, we now turn to the estimation of r_H^*, the other essential parameter to carry out GRACE calculations.

The key idea goes back to the general formula in Eq. (8.3b), repeated here for convenience:

$$r_H^* = 1 - \omega_H - \varepsilon^{\omega_H} \tag{8.14}$$

This means that knowing r_H^* requires knowing both ω_H and how it changes with H (quantified in the form of the elasticity ε^{ω_H}).

We begin with Eq. (8.12) and take the derivative of that with respect to H, giving $\dfrac{\partial \omega_H}{\partial H} = \dfrac{\beta_2}{H}$. From this,

$$\varepsilon^{\omega_H}(H) = \frac{\partial \omega_H}{\partial H}\left(\frac{H}{\omega_H}\right) = \frac{\beta_2}{\omega_H} = \frac{\beta_2}{\beta_1 + \beta_2 \ln(H)} \tag{8.15a}$$

or in the empirical estimation form,

$$\widehat{\varepsilon^{\omega_H}} = \frac{\widehat{\beta_2}}{\widehat{\omega_H}} = \frac{\widehat{\beta_2}}{\widehat{\beta_1} + \widehat{\beta_2} \ln(H)} \tag{8.15b}$$

With this estimate, using Eq. (8.14), we now can estimate r_H^*, along with the ways in which each parameter varies with H. Their variability with H hinges on β_2 in the happiness equation, which determines if there is any "curvature" in the relationship between $\ln(\text{Happiness})$ and $\ln(H)$. If $\beta_2 = 0$, then $\varepsilon^{\omega_H} = 0$, and our GRACE world is greatly simplified. But, as we discussed in Chapter 2, it is quite important to know if r_H^* is constant or not, so this complete estimation approach can be quite valuable.

Putting all of the pieces together, our final estimate of r_H^* becomes

$$\widehat{r_H^*}(H) = 1 - \hat{\omega}_H(H) - \widehat{\varepsilon^\omega}(H) = 1 - (\hat{\beta}_1 + \hat{\beta}_2 \ln(H)) - \frac{\hat{\beta}_2}{\hat{\beta}_1 + \hat{\beta}_2 \ln(H)}$$

(8.16a)

Again, if $\hat{\beta}_2 = 0$, this simplifies to

$$\widehat{r_H^*}(H) = 1 - \hat{\omega}_H(H) = 1 - \widehat{\beta}_1 \qquad (8.16b)$$

Finally, we can provide an empirical estimate of γ by combining our Happiness-based estimates of ω_H and r_H^* using Eq. (8.7b), repeated here for convenience:

$$\hat{\gamma} = \frac{\widehat{\omega_H}}{\widehat{\omega_H} + \widehat{r_H^*}} \qquad (8.17)$$

Using Eq. (8.8a), once we know $\hat{\gamma}$ and $\widehat{r^*}$, we have an estimate of Δ, which permits estimates of the higher order risk preference terms required in GRACE, a task to which we turn next.

Extending Results to Additional GRACE Parameters Using HARA Utility

We can now return to some of the many benefits of assuming HARA utility. We have now shown how to estimate ω_H, r_H^*, and γ using results from happiness regression models. Using the results from the previous section on the HARA utility function, we can now readily see how to build up to higher level risk parameters with no further estimation needed. The key goes back to Eqs. (8.8a) and (8.8b). Once we know r_H^* in the HARA model, then $\pi_H^* = r_H^* + \Delta$, $\tau_H^* = \pi_H^* + \Delta$, and so forth for all necessary higher order risk terms.

Estimating Key GRACE Parameters

We can now review each of these key GRACE calculations. From Chapter 2, the first is the adjustment to K, the standard cost-effectiveness analysis (CEA) threshold. That adjustment is

$$\omega_H R = \omega_H \left\{ 1 + r_H^* \ell^* + \frac{1}{2} r_H^* \pi_H^* \ell^{*2} + \frac{1}{6} r_H^* \pi_H^* \tau_H^* \ell^{*3} + \ldots \right\} \tag{8.18}$$

This formula uses the Taylor series expansion around untreated illness severity, ℓ^*. We obtain ω_H from the happiness model using Eq. (8.12), r_H^* from Eq. (8.16a), and the higher order risk terms as discussed in the section on the HARA utility function and in the immediately preceding section.

The second adjustment to traditional CEA arises when calculating the disability adjustment to WTP. Recall that in Chapter 5, we introduced the disability-adjusting factor ψ, so that

$$K_{\text{GRACE}}^D = \frac{K \omega_H R}{1 - \psi d^*} \tag{8.19}$$

The factor ψ is also a Taylor series expansion, except this time, it is centered around the level of disability in the baseline state, d^*:

$$\psi \equiv \omega_H \left(1 + \frac{1}{2} r_H^* d^* + \frac{1}{6} r_H^* \pi_H^* (d^*)^2 + \frac{1}{24} r_H^* \pi_H^* \tau_H^* d^3 \ldots \right) \tag{8.20}$$

The estimation of ψ takes place in the same way, using estimates of the risk parameters and ω_H just as in the computation of R. The only difference is that the risk parameters should be evaluated at d^* rather than ℓ^*, the proper point of departure when estimating R. The happiness model provides mechanisms to adjust ω_H and r_H^* as necessary if utility is not CRRA, and all other higher order terms follow immediately.

The third occasion upon which this occurs comes during the estimation of the marginal rate of substitution between HRQoL and LE, as discussed in Chapter 4. There, we needed to estimate the factor ρ, which helps measure how that trade-off (marginal rate of substitution) varies with severity of *treated* illness. The Taylor Series approximation is given by

$$\rho = 1 - \omega_H \left[t^* + \frac{1}{2} r_H^* t^{*2} + \frac{1}{6} r_H^* \pi_H^* t^{*3} + \frac{1}{24} r_H^* \pi_H^* \tau_H^* \ell^* t^{*4} \ldots \right] \qquad (8.21)$$

Here, the risk terms are evaluated (respectively) around t^* and d^*, which may again require adjustment to the estimated values of r_H^* and ω_H using the information from the happiness estimates, unless utility is CRRA, in which case no adjustment is needed.

This same symmetry carries over to the risk adjustment for quality-adjusted life years, which takes into account the variability of treatment outcomes (see Chapter 3). As shown in Eq. (3.1), that adjustment factor is

$$\varepsilon \approx 1 + \left[\frac{\mu_H}{\mu_B} \right] \left[\begin{array}{c} -\frac{1}{2} r_H^* \left(\frac{1}{\mu_H} \right)^2 \Delta \sigma_H^2 + \frac{1}{6} \pi_H^* r_H^* \left(\frac{1}{\mu_H} \right)^3 \Delta \left[\gamma_1 \sigma_H^3 \right] \\ -\frac{1}{24} \tau_H^* \pi_H^* r_H^* \left(\frac{1}{\mu_H} \right)^2 \Delta \left[\gamma_2 \sigma_H^4 \right] \ldots \end{array} \right] \qquad (8.22)$$

In this case (as in the estimation of R), these risk-preference parameters should be evaluated at the level of untreated health, $H = H_0(1 - \ell^*)$. Again, the happiness model provides direct ways to do this.

These calculations are simplified considerably if the risk parameters do not vary with H. If we have CRRA utility, then ω_H, r_H^*, π_H^* and τ_H^* (and all higher order terms) will have the same value at all levels of H. But this may not be true. Fortunately, the happiness economics model allows us to understand whether or not we have CRRA. It is simply an econometric test as to whether $\beta_2 = 0$ in the happiness regression, as shown in Eq. (8.11).

Having completed our discussion of the happiness economics method, we now turn to another widely used approach to estimating risk parameters—the discrete choice experiment (DCE) method.

ESTIMATION USING DISCRETE CHOICE EXPERIMENTS

Discrete choice experiments provide a well-understood way to estimate people's attitudes toward risk. We begin with the relatively simple task of estimating people's risk aversion, from which we can build toward estimation of higher order risk parameters. This approach requires that the researcher assume a specific form of the utility function, but once that choice is made, the process is fairly straightforward. Readers will note that the DCE and happiness methods do not begin with the same parameter estimates for GRACE because they approach the estimation problem from different perspectives. Happiness methods end up estimating ω_H and r_H^*. DCE methods, as we shall see, instead estimate r_H^* and π_H^*. Nevertheless, they can both lead to the same end point due to the assumptions built into the HARA utility function methodology.

Estimating Relative Risk Aversion

The basic concept of DCE is built on the economic concept of "indifference," only instead of the simple indifference curves used in Chapter 2, we have to use some math because the concepts resolve around "indifference" between gambles that involve probabilities. We begin with the concept of a certainty equivalent (CE). The CE is a fixed sum of money (obtained with 100% probability) that a person views as having the same value as a gamble involving uncertain outcomes. Suppose that the gamble is structured so that you receive x_1 in your favorite currency (dollars, euros, yen, yuan, pounds sterling, bitcoins, etc.) with probability p and x_2 with probability $(1 - p)$. The expected *payoff*, of course, is simply $E(x) = px_1 + (1 - p)x_2$. But if people are risk averse, then the value in any given state is not the actual amount of money but, rather, the utility of that amount of money. Therefore, the expected utility of the same gamble is

$$E(U) = pU(x_1) + (1 - p)U(x_2) \tag{8.23}$$

The CE is the "certain" amount of money that the person would willingly exchange for the (risky) proceeds of the gamble. Therefore, the CE is the amount of money such that $U(CE) = E(U)$, as shown in Eq. (8.23). This structure allows estimation of the degree of risk aversion, once the researcher assumes a specific utility function.

Partly because it is widely used, and partly because it is relatively simple to analyze, we proceed initially by using the CRRA utility function of the form $U(x) = x^{1-\gamma}$. It is easy to show that this utility function has constant relative risk aversion, where $r^* = \gamma$. When $\gamma = 0$ (no risk aversion), then utility is linear in x. With this simple CRRA function, the expected utility of a simple gamble is

$$E(U) = p\left[x_1^{1-\gamma}\right] + (1-p)\left[x_2^{1-\gamma}\right] \tag{8.24}$$

Now consider a person with a risk aversion level of $\gamma = 0.5$ and confronted with a gamble that paid \$10,000 with probability $p = 0.3$ and \$100 with probability $(1 - p) = 0.7$, so $E(x) = \$3070$. A risk-neutral person is indifferent between this gamble and its expected value. However, the point of indifference will be lower for a risk-averse person, as we can demonstrate using the CRRA utility function.[11] With a risk aversion level of 0.5, the expected utility of this gamble is

$$E(U) = 0.3[\$10,000^{0.5}] + 0.7[100^{0.5}] = .3[100] + .7[10] = 37 \tag{8.25}$$

In contrast, the utility value of the average payoff is $3070^{0.5} = 55.41$. Therefore, a rational person with this level of risk aversion would always prefer to take the average payoff for sure, instead of the gamble itself, because 55.41 exceeds 37.

This leads us to the CE. With this level of risk aversion, what amount of cash provides the same level of utility as the gamble? The answer is \$1,369 because $U(\$1369) = 1369^{0.5} = 37$ when utility is CRRA and the relative risk aversion parameter is $\gamma = 0.5$.

To explore this further, if γ is only 0.1 (rather than 0.5), a much lower level of relative risk aversion, the expected utility of the gamble is

$0.3(\$10,000^{0.9}) + 0.7(100^{0.9}) \approx 1238.49$. The certain amount of money providing the same level of utility (the CE) is found by solving $x^{0.9} = \$1238.49$. That value is $x = \$2732.42$, still lower than (but much closer to) the average value of the gamble, \$3,070. To further reduce the level, if $\gamma = 0.01$, a trivial level of relative risk aversion, then the CE is \$3,037, almost the same as the expected value of the gamble, \$3,070.

We can solve this same problem in reverse. Supposing that some people tell us that for the gamble just discussed, the maximum they would willingly pay to "roll the dice" is \$2,500. From that, we can discern their degree of relative risk aversion by finding the level of γ in the equation to make the CE equal to \$2,500. The answer turns out to be (rounding slightly) $r_C^* = \gamma = 0.167$.

To further explore this problem, if the maximum WTP to participate in the gamble was stated as \$1,500, then the solution value is approximately to choose a specific CE, $\gamma = 0.46$. Going even further, if the WTP to participate in the gamble (the CE) was only \$500, that would indicate a very high degree of relative risk aversion, with $r^* \approx 0.9$. Higher levels of relative risk aversion always lead to lower levels of WTP to engage in the gamble.

In a classic study on this topic, Holt and Laury (2002) did something quite similar. But instead of asking respondents to specific CE, they asked them to choose among pairs of gambles, each of which had the same amounts of money [like x_1 and x_2 in Eqs. (8.23) and (8.24)], but which varied the probabilities of the outcomes [like p in Eqs. (8.23) and (8.24)]. The choices are set up so that Option A has much less risk (the gap between the payments is only \$0.40), whereas Option B is much riskier (the gap is \$3.75). Therefore, risk-averse people should opt for Option A until the extra *expected* earnings of Option B flip their decision by adding enough to the expected payoff to overcome the economic loss due to uncertainty. As the gap in expected payoffs between B and A increases (see the last column in Table 8.1), most risk-averse people will eventually flip to Option B, but the more risk averse they are, the further down the table they would wait before flipping to Option B. The two gambles that "surround" their "flipping points" (the last gamble where A is chosen and the first gamble where B is chosen) put boundaries on the range of risk aversion parameters where the person is "nearly indifferent" using calculations such as Eq. (8.24). Their table of gambles offered to respondents is shown in Table 8.1.

Respondents were asked to choose Option A or Option B for each of the 10 gambles, and as you work your way down Table 8.1, the probability of the higher outcome increases. The last row, in fact, is a "no brainer" because the subjects get $3.85 for sure by choosing Option B versus $2.00 by choosing Option A. It was included as a test of respondents' rationality.

Table 8.2 shows the results for the "low-stakes" gamble shown in Table 8.1 and also for a "hypothetical" high-stakes gamble (20X the payoffs), and a real 20X stakes gamble, where the money was quite significant (the respondents were mostly college students). The latter two experiments test to determine if "hypothetical" and "actual" payoffs yield different results. We discuss this issue in a subsequent section.

The first column of Table 8.2 shows the number of "safe choices"—that is, choosing Option A, which has the much lower risk. The second column shows the degree of relative risk aversion implied by the choices, using the same general approach as that shown in Eq. (8.25). For example, if the respondents switched from Option A to Option B after five safe choices,

Table 8.1 TEN PAIRED LOTTERY CHOICE DECISIONS WITH LOW-VALUE PAYOFFS

Option A	Option B	Expected Payoff Difference
1/10 of $2.00, 9/10 of $1.60	1/10 of $3.85, 9/10 of $0.10	$1.17
2/10 of $2.00, 8/10 of $1.60	2/10 of $3.85, 8/10 of $0.10	$0.83
3/10 of $2.00, 7/10 of $1.60	3/10 of $3.85, 7/10 of $0.10	$0.50
4/10 of $2.00, 6/10 of $1.60	4/10 of $3.85, 6/10 of $0.10	$0.16
5/10 of $2.00, 5/10 of $1.60	5/10 of $3.85, 5/10 of $0.10	−$0.18
6/10 of $2.00, 4/10 of $1.60	6/10 of $3.85, 4/10 of $0.10	−$0.51
7/10 of $2.00, 3/10 of $1.60	7/10 of $3.85, 3/10 of $0.10	−$0.85
8/10 of $2.00, 2/10 of $1.60	8/10 of $3.85, 2/10 of $0.10	−$0.18
9/10 of $2.00, 1/10 of $1.60	9/10 of $3.85, 1/10 of $0.10	−$0.52
10/10 of $2.00, 0/10 of $1.60	10/10 of $3.85, 0/10 of $0.10	−$0.85

Reproduced from Holt and Laury (2002).

Table 8.2 Risk Aversion Classification Based on Lottery Choices

No. of Safe Choices	Range of Relative Risk Aversion for $U(X1 - r/(1 - r)$	Risk Preference Classification	Proportion of Choices		
			Low Real[a]	High Real	High Hypothetical
0–1	$r < -0.95$	Highly risk loving	.01	.01	.03
2	$-0.95 < r < -0.49$	Very risk loving	.01	.01	.04
3	$-0.95 < r < -0.15$	Risk loving	.06	.04	.08
4	$-0.15 < r < 0.15$	Risk neural	.26	.13	.29
5	$0.15 < r < 0.41$	Slightly risk averse	.26	.19	.16
6	$0.41 < r < 0.68$	Risk averse	.23	.23	.25
7	$0.68 < r < 0.97$	Very risk averse	.13	.22	.09
8	$0.97 < r < 1.37$	Highly risk averse	.03	.11	.03
9–10	$1.37 < r$	Stay in bed	.01	.06	

[a] Average over first and second decisions.

Reproduced from Holt and Laury (2002).

it means that the fifth gamble has an implicit relative risk aversion of $r^* = 0.15$ and the sixth gamble has an implicit risk aversion of $r^* = 0.41$. These choices place boundaries on the degree of risk aversion each respondent has by looking where the switch from Option A to Option B occurred. Obviously, one can shrink the boundaries in this approach by offering respondents more gambles from which to choose but narrower gaps between adjacent gamble structures. This trades off precision of estimation versus respondent burden. Even in conducting research, life is full of trade-offs!

You can see several things from Table 8.2. First, almost all of the respondents exhibited risk-averse behavior. The "median" degree of risk aversion was "slightly risk averse" in the "low stakes, real" experiment, and it rose to "risk averse" in the "high stakes, real" experiment. In the "hypothetical, high" experiment, the median degree of risk aversion was "slightly risk averse," lower than appeared when "real money" was at stake. This suggests that hypothetical gambles elicit different and, in this case, less risk averse responses than when "the real deal" is at stake. We return to this issue when assessing how this might affect DCE experiments to assess risk aversion in health, because such studies will almost certainly involve hypothetical, not "real," differences in health outcomes.

Noussair et al. (2014) use a slightly different method to estimate relative risk aversion. They offer respondents two options, labeled "Left" and "Right." Instead of asking respondents to compare two gambles, their Left option is a fixed number (€20, €25, €35, or €40) and the Right option is a gamble involving outcomes of either €65 or €5, so their approach directly matches Eq. (8.25). Differently than in Holt and Laury (2002), Noussair et al. keep all of the probabilities the same (50–50 odds) but vary the financial stakes. Either approach suffices to estimate relative risk aversion. Noussair et al. also use two different formulas to represent the utility of various amounts of money to measuring relative risk parameters in their population. Their first model, using CRRA, found $r_C^* = 0.88$, $\pi_C^* = 1.88$, and $\tau_C^* = 2.88$, separated by 1.0, as the CRRA model requires. Using a more flexible utility function, the expo-power as developed by Saha (1993), they estimated $r_C^* = 0.93$, $\pi_C^* = 1.68$ and $\tau_C^* = 2.58$. These values suggest (see Eq. 8.9a) that utility in money is IRRA, since $(\pi_C^* - r_C^*) < 1$.

Estimating Relative Prudence

Having gone through the estimation of relative risk aversion, the next step is relatively straightforward. Noussair et al. (2014), show that in order to estimate higher order risk preferences, researchers must present compound gambles to respondents rather than the simple gambles needed to assess relative risk aversion. Their Figure 1, reproduced here as Figure 8.2, shows the necessary types of gambles to estimate relative prudence.

In Noussair et al.'s (2014) Figure 1, Lotteries L ("left") and R ("right") have one gamble choosing between x and y, but then a subsequent gamble appears, involving either the addition or the subtraction of a separate amount z. In Lottery L, this second gamble comes if outcome x happens,

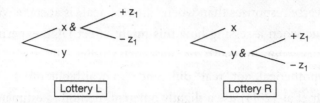

Figure 8.2 Risk apportionment task identifying prudence.
Reproduced from Noussair et al. (2010).

and in Lottery R, the second gamble (involving z) happens only after outcome y happens.

The lotteries in Noussair et al.'s (2014) Figure 1 had the following structure in their experiments: The Left lottery primarily used $x = $ €90 and $y = $ €60. Then z was varied between €10 and €40 with random presentation of the order of choices with different values of z. Obviously, as z rises, the degree of risk rises. The Right lottery primarily used $x = $ €90 and $y = $ €60, with z again varying between €10 and €40.[12] Although the probability structure is more complicated, the same conceptual idea is involved, where the expected utility of the gamble depends on the risk aversion, and the switching point between Left and Right indicates the subjects' relative prudence, which basically determines how fast (if at all) relative risk aversion changes as (in their experiments) income changes. The Left lottery has the added variance only after the €90 outcome has occurred, whereas the Right lottery does the same thing after the lower (y) outcome of €60 has occurred. When subjects choose one or the other, they reveal how their risk preferences change with income. Researchers can then acquire additional information by varying the amount of risk, accomplished simply by altering the magnitude of z.

Other Risk and Preference Parameters

The combination of these two experiments—one to measure relative risk aversion, r_C^*, and one to measure relative prudence, π_C^*—provides sufficient information to carry out the entire GRACE modeling structure. The same logical structure should allow estimation of the comparable health risk parameters, r_H^* and π_H^*.

Estimation of ω_H in the DCE environment simply requires estimates of r_H^* and γ. As shown previously, in HARA utility, $\omega_H = \left[\dfrac{\gamma}{1-\gamma}\right] r_H^*$. As first shown by Phelps and Cinatl (2021), knowing r_H^* and π_H^* allows estimation of γ (see Eq. 8.6), thereby allowing estimation of ω_H. All of the higher order risk terms can be estimated using Δ as described in previously.

Because of the parameter linkages provided by assuming HARA utility (the Δ term), we envision no need to estimate directly the higher order parameters such as relative temperance (τ_H^*) using DCE methods, even though it is possible (using increasingly complex gambles presented to research subjects). This creates a parsimony of research effort within the DCE structure that eliminates the need for increasingly complex gambles presented to respondents, thus minimizing respondent burden and researcher effort.

Furthermore, Eq. (8.8b) allows the analyst to evaluate all these risk preference terms at any desired level of health. Due to HARA utility, a DCE measuring just two parameters, r_H^* and π_H^*, evaluated at a single level of health can be used to estimate all of GRACE's risk preference parameters at any desired level of HRQoL.

As previous studies (c.f., Holt and Laury, 2002; Noussair et al., 2014) have shown, estimating the key risk parameters, r_H^* and π_H^*, requires fitting the gamble/choice data using maximum likelihood estimation (MLE) methods to recover the relevant utility function parameters from the subjects' responses. Equation (8.25) shows one such equation for the isoelastic (CRRA) utility function that only has one parameter to estimate.

Both Holt and Laury (2002) and Noussair et al. (2014) fitted their data both to CRRA utility (one parameter) and to Expo-Power utility (two parameters) using MLE techniques (see Appendix 8.1).

Our suggestion to others pursuing such research would have them fit the data to HARA utility functions, also requiring two parameters (γ and b), thus directly providing the necessary parameters to complete the portfolio of new risk-preference parameters required by GRACE.

Exact GRACE Models Versus Taylor Series Approximations

We again refer readers to Appendix 6.1 regarding "exact utility" representations of the TVMI in the GRACE model. Estimation of utility parameters using DCE methods requires that analysts assume a specific utility function such as CRRA, HARA, or expo-power. Once these models are estimated, the exact model for GRACE is simple to implement by using the assumed functional form and its estimated parameters to replace $W(H)$ and $W'(H)$ as needed. When values such as ρ require estimation of expected utility values, the simple average of the estimated utilities for each observed patient suffices, since expected utility theory tells us that value is linear in utility itself.

Hypothetical Versus Real DCE Choices

The question naturally arises as to whether hypothetical gambles can elicit meaningful responses from research subjects that would match their responses if "real" gambles were involved. When studying financial outcomes, it is of course easy to compare real and hypothetical responses as long as the research project has a sufficiently large budget to pay off the gambles chosen by the subjects. In the realm of health care, however, the use of real gambles would be ethically prohibited, and so it is of interest to know what has been learned in the study of real versus hypothetical gambles in the realm of money.

Noussair et al. (2014) specifically tested hypothetical gambles versus real gambles with actual euro payments attached to them. They call these "real" experiments "incentivized." They report specifically that

> . . . there are no significant differences between the Real and the [Hypothetical] treatments for any of the measures. This suggests that non-incentivised choices provide unbiased estimates of the average attitudes of a population for similar risks and real stakes. . . . The results support the view that hypothetical lottery questions are

a valid, unbiased instrument to elicit risk attitudes on survey panels where real financial incentives cannot be implemented (p. 335).

Holt and Laury (2002) also tested for real versus hypothetical gambles and found that the real gambles produced higher estimates of risk aversion than appeared in the hypothetical tests. Table 8.2 shows their results.

We believe that the "body of evidence" suggests that hypothetical gambles may be unbiased compared to real gambles, but this issue is far from certain, and the relationship may vary from case to case. In any event, we envision no realistic alternative to using hypothetical gambles involving health outcomes because we believe it would be difficult to get institutional review boards to authorize experiments that randomly inflicted real and differing levels of health outcomes on participants.[13] Thus, DCE estimation of risk preferences in health will almost certainly rely on respondents' choices among hypothetical situations.

SUMMARY

Our review of research methods suggests that either happiness models or DCE models could be used to measure risk attitudes in H. Neither method is ideal—both have potential flaws—but if we are to proceed with the implementation of GRACE, some estimates of ω_H, r_H^* and π_H^* must be made, as well as (desirably) knowing how these parameters change over different levels of H (or, alternatively, knowing that they are constant across H). Regardless of the method chosen, the researcher needs only to estimate r_H^* and π_H^* for one particular level of H. The HARA utility framework can then be used to infer all other risk preference parameters used by GRACE and even to evaluate all these parameters at any other relevant level of H.

Although we have not carried out any estimation of these parameters, we hope that perhaps some readers of this book will be spurred by the ideas herein and create new estimates of the key risk preferences in health. We welcome all such efforts—the more, the merrier!

Putting Together the Parts

The whole is greater than the sum of the parts.

—ARISTOTLE (*Metaphysics*, Book 8)

INTRODUCTION AND "WORK PLAN"

To date, we know of no studies that fully implement the generalized risk-adjusted cost-effectiveness (GRACE) model. The key missing data involve an understanding of the degree of risk aversion in HRQoL, how it might change across levels of health, and also how rapidly returns to HRQoL decline as the level of HRQoL grows from 0 (the worst possible health state) to 1 (the best imaginable health state).

To implement GRACE, we need estimates of ω_H, r_H^*, π_H^*, which then imply estimates of all higher order risk parameters (for details, see Chapter 8). These will soon be available in the literature, but they are not yet published as of the time of writing.

In parallel, almost all studies comparing medical interventions, whether randomized controlled trials (RCTs), comparative effectiveness studies (e.g., undertaken or sponsored by the Patient-Centered Outcomes Research Institute), or others, report only average treatment outcomes (and their differences). They conduct statistical tests to determine if these differences are "real," but they seldom, if ever, report differences in the variances (and in skewness and kurtosis, if present) of outcomes. Instead,

Valuing Health. Charles E. Phelps and Darius N. Lakdawalla, Oxford University Press. © Oxford University Press 2024.
DOI: 10.1093/oso/9780197686287.003.0009

such studies commonly report "p values" that derive from prespecified levels of the probability that the outcome appears by chance (e.g., 5% or 1%). These data are insufficient to calculate the actual variances of the outcomes in the treatment (T) and comparison (C) arms of the clinical studies. GRACE requires the actual variance measures and, in addition, measures of skewness and (desirably) kurtosis.

Because of these current data limitations, we can only present a hypothetical model of how to assemble a GRACE analysis. In this example, we use a single period from the multiperiod model developed in Chapter 6. The full model, repeated here from Eq. (6.2a), satisfies

$$\text{NMB}_0 = \phi \sum_{n=1}^{N} \beta^n \{[KD\omega_H R_n][\mu_{pn}\delta_n + p_n^U \mu_{Bn}\varepsilon_n] - (p_n^U \Delta C_n + \mu_p C_n^T)\} \quad (9.1a)$$

Because the calculation of costs is a standard part of CEA and not modified by GRACE, we focus instead on the actual monetary benefit (MB) viewed from the perspective of period 0, ignoring costs. Because the discounting factor β^n does not differ from standard cost-effectiveness analysis (CEA) and, indeed, cost–benefit analysis models, we set that aside here also, concentrating on the per-period benefit, repeated from Eq. (6.1.d):

$$\text{Per-period benefit} = [K\omega_H R_n D_n \phi][\mu_{pn}\delta_n + p_n^U \mu_{Bn}\varepsilon_n] \quad (9.1b)$$

Finally, to avoid notational clutter, we drop the n subscripts everywhere. Recall that p^U is the untreated probability of survival from period 0 to period n and that ϕ is the probability of contracting the disease in period 1. Setting $\phi = 1$ and $p_n^U = 1$ allows us to adopt an ex post perspective on the GRACE method of measuring benefits. Generalization to the full model is relatively simple. With this series of simplifications, we have

$$\text{One period value} = [K\omega_H RD][\mu_p \delta + \mu_B \varepsilon] \quad (9.1c)$$

Equation (9.1c) further can be broken into two parts, which we separately analyze. The first part defines the willingness to pay (WTP) for health gains, which we call K_{GRACE}^D. It is defined in its fullest complexity as $K_{GRACE}^D = KD\omega_H R$. This is the complete way to measure value because of the effect of diminishing returns to H, captured in ω_H; the effects of illness severity, R; and the effect of existing permanent disability, D. The second part of Eq. (9.1c) measures the "effective" and "risk-adjusted" gain in health, $[\mu_p\delta + \phi p\mu_B\varepsilon]$.

As Chapter 4 developed, because GRACE, like almost all other health economics analyses, assumes linear utility in life expectancy (LE), we can also use the proof that $\delta = \dfrac{\rho H_0}{\omega_H R}$, so that

$$\text{One period value} = KD\{\rho H_0\mu_p\} + K_{GRACE}^D\{\mu_B\varepsilon\} \qquad (9.1d)$$

Since $K_{GRACE}^D = K\omega_H RD$, this emphasizes that the effects of diminishing returns on value, $\omega_H R$, only apply to mean gains in HRQoL as adjusted for effects of uncertain treatment outcomes, $\mu_B\varepsilon$.

Our focus at this point is the measurements of ω_H and R, the latter of which requires estimation of the risk-preference parameters r_H^*, π_H^*, and τ_H^*, as well as the severity of untreated disease, ℓ^*. These are the key elements that distinguish GRACE from standard CEA. We return in a later section of this chapter to discuss the issues arising when permanent disability enters the model. We again remind the reader that the exact utility version of GRACE bypasses the Taylor series approximations that require higher-order risk preference terms, as Appendix 6.1 details.

The average gains in LE and HRQoL, μ_p and μ_B, are identical to those used in standard CEA. The remaining components of Eq. (9.1d) require estimation of D, ρ, and ε, recalling, of course, that the latter two are period-specific in the full multiperiod model.

Now, focus on the "average difference" in treatment effects for HRQoL, μ_B, which represents the typical measure of gain in standard CEA studies such as RCTs or comparative effectiveness studies. In GRACE, that average value must be multiplied by the risk-adjustment factor, ε to account for uncertainty in treatment outcomes. Chapter 3 discusses these issues.

Treatment can also include improvements in survival probability, the average of which is measured by μ_p (per period). To be commensurate with gains in HRQoL (so we can add them together), we must also convert LE gains into "equivalent" HRQoL gains through use of δ, the marginal rate of substitution (MRS) between LE and HRQoL, which we estimate using $\dfrac{\rho H_0}{\omega_H R}$. Standard CEA assumes that this trade-off rate is the same at all levels of HRQoL, but when we introduce diminishing returns to HRQoL, that also means that the trade-off rate $\dfrac{\rho H_0}{\omega_H R}$ varies with measurements of risk a version in H. Chapter 4 discusses these issues.

We will show how to estimate each of these component parts to complete a full GRACE measure of value. That "benefit," multiplied by the WTP per unit of benefit, K^D_{GRACE}, provides the total measure of value in GRACE. The risk-preference parameters, $\omega_H, r^*_H, \pi^*_H, \tau^*_H$, only need to be measured "once," not with every health technology assessment (HTA) effort. These risk-preference parameters are then combined with data from RCTs or other HTA studies that measure burden of disability and both untreated and treated illness, d^*, ℓ^*, and t^*. Combining these two types of data provides the basis for estimating key parameters in Eq. (9.1d), including D, R, ρ, and ε. We can then assemble them into the final GRACE value measures and repeat them as needed using period-specific parameter values. Alternatively, using the "exact" form of GRACE as elaborated in Appendix 6.1, one only needs estimates of any specific utility function's parameters.

MEASURING HEALTH OUTCOMES IN GRACE

Measurement Tools

At several different steps, GRACE requires measures of health levels of affected individuals—in the untreated (acute illness) state, the treated (acute illness) state, or without acute illness but with a preexisting disability. We measure the proportional losses from perfect health in these three states as ℓ^*, t^*, and d^*, respectively. Each is measured on an index of HRQoL that ranges from 0 = worst possible HRQoL health status to 1 = best imaginable HRQoL health state. We now turn to methods to measure these HRQoL levels.

In GRACE, the primary measure of health outcomes is stated in a summary measure of the levels of health enjoyed by patients at various levels of illness (healthy, disabled but not diseased, untreated disease, and treated disease levels), often referred to as the HRQoL adjustment used to calculate a quality-adjusted life year (QALY). The specific mechanism to measure HRQoL is not central to our example. The only requirement is that the measures correspond to *levels of health*, not the utilities thereof. Without endorsing it specifically, we next summarize how one such health status index is constructed to provide clarity on the type of measure that GRACE requires.[1]

An Example

The Patient Reported Outcomes Measurement Information System (PROMIS), developed by the U.S. National Institutes of Health (NIH), provides an example of health status measuring systems that would work in the GRACE model. One of the most widely used and general metrics (PROMIS Global-10) measures health in 10 dimensions: (1) general health; (2) quality of life; (3) physical health; (4) mental health; (5) satisfaction with social activities; (6) ability to carry out everyday activities; (7) pain; (8) fatigue; (9) ability to carry out usual roles and activities; and (10) frequency of being anxious, depressed, or irritable in past week.

Each of these dimensions (or "domains") of HRQoL is measured on a 5-point scale. In most cases, this converts five word-based answers (poor, fair, good, very good, and excellent) into a 5-point numerical scale. A few domains have reversed measurement, so, for example, the 10th question measures "how often" the mental health issues occur, with "always" rated 1, up to "never" rated 5. "Pain" is collapsed from a score of 10 (worst pain imaginable) to 0 (no pain) so that increasingly low responses on the pain scale are converted into increasingly higher (better) scores on the standard 1–5 scale used throughout PROMIS.

The Global-10 sums the responses with specific weighting using item response theory (IRT) methods.[2] This method, for example, gives more weight to a task that is more difficult (e.g., walking 1 mile vs. getting out of bed). It also uses item discrimination methods to increase the precision of the final score. Aside from these IRT weighting modifications, Global-10 is a linear sum of the numerical values assigned to the responses to the 10 questions.

The PROMIS system provides more detailed measurement of specific aspects of health, which can then be combined into the more general concepts shown in the top half of Figure 9.1, the representation of the PROMIS system provided by NIH. The lower half of this figure shows some of the additional and more specific measures of health status that PROMIS can provide. Some of these can be collected together in

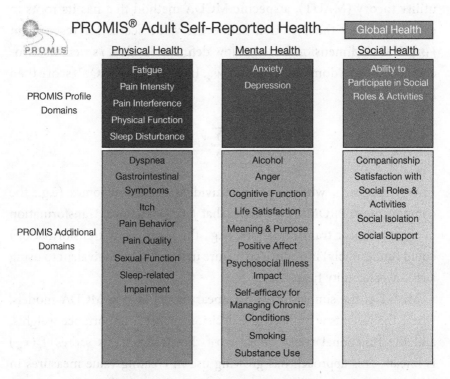

Figure 9.1 NIH representation of the different dimensions of health that PROMIS can measure.

composite form to provide higher level measures, such as those involving "pain."

WEIGHTING THE HEALTH DOMAINS

Except for the IRT adjustments, PROMIS simply adds the scores of the 10 health domains. In concept, one could assign "importance weights" to each domain of health. In some sense, these relative values represent utility preferences, but they do not convey any information about diminishing returns to health—the key requirement for our desired HRQoL measurement. They simply provide a mechanism to add the individual "attribute" scores (domains of health) together in a weighted (rather than unweighted) fashion.

The methods to combine multiple items into a single measure of value are well known, generally characterized as multi-criteria decision analysis (MCDA). We provide an example using multi-attribute utility theory (MAUT), a specific MCDA method that has its roots in expected utility theory. First, define the value scores for respondent j on HRQoL dimension k as x_{jk}. Now define individual j's weights associated with each domain of value as w_{jk}. Individual j's HRQoL score then becomes

$$\mathrm{HRQoL}_j = \sum_k w_{jk} f_k(x_{jk}) \qquad (9.2)$$

In our approach, where x_{jk} are individual health outcomes (e.g., the components of PROMIS), we desire that $f_k(x_{jk})$ is a linear transformation of x_{jk}. Nonlinear transformations (e.g., the logarithmic transformation) could (undesirably) introduce curvature that would be equivalent to using a risk-averse utility function.

MAUT is the simplest possible linear model among MCDA models, where the weights w_{jk} reflect "the decision-maker's" importance weights, and the functional transformation of the health status scores $f_k(x_{jk})$ is linear.[3] This approach has growing use in creating value measures in health care (Phelps and Madhavan, 2017; Phelps et al., 2018).

Unambiguously, whether weighted by MAUT methods or not, PROMIS does not estimate the *utility* of health levels but, rather, measures the *level* of health that can readily be converted into the 0–1 scale required by GRACE. It measures "HRQoL" in the sense that we intend—a measure of health status. Thus, PROMIS provides a useful example of the type of health status measurement that GRACE requires.

INTERMEDIATE HEALTH OUTCOMES

We note here that some medical interventions use intermediate outcomes to measure a therapy's performance, a practice that can help in comparing treatments within the same disease category but which is not sufficient for use in GRACE. In GRACE, gains in LE and HRQoL must be combined using the estimated value for the MRS between these two dimensions of health. The simple reason is that no common measures exist of WTP for all these various intermediate outcomes. Furthermore, it is not possible to compare the value of treatments across different disorders when intermediate outcomes are used. Therefore, in order to use intermediate outcome measures, researchers must find a valid link between the intermediate outcome and the final health outcome (Jonas et al., 2018).

Mean Treatment Outcome Measurements

Standard CEA requires measurement of average treatment effects, both for HRQoL improvements (μ_B) and for improvements in LE measured as improvements in the probability of survival into the subsequent period (μ_P). GRACE requires that μ_B be measured using a health status measuring system such as PROMIS. Any measurement system suffices as long as it measures health status, not the utility thereof.

These simple measurements of health gains, μ_B and μ_P, are the primary focus of standard HTA analyses and clinical studies that support them (e.g., RCTs or comparative effectiveness studies). But to combine them in GRACE to the full measure of health gain as shown in Eq. (9.1d), we need to estimate the risk-preference values embedded in GRACE. We turn next to developing the key components of $K^D_{\text{GRACE}} = KD\omega_H R$.

UNIQUE COMPONENTS OF K^D_{GRACE}

Our "plan of action" is to select some (completely arbitrary) values of the necessary parameters (as if they had been previously estimated) and then assemble these data into a single, specific measure of benefit using GRACE. We emphasize, however, that this exercise is only intended to show how to "put all the pieces together," and in no way do we intend this to represent a "typical" GRACE outcome. Chapter 8 discussed at length two ways to estimate these risk-preference parameters. Our discussion here presumes that good estimates of those parameters have emerged from such studies, and we employ them here.

Calculating the Severity of Illness Adjustment Factor R

In addition to the risk-preference values that Chapter 8 discusses, the next datum needed is the illness severity measure, ℓ^*. Values of ℓ^* have commonly been determined in previous CEA studies and are widely cataloged in the Tufts University CEVR database, which now includes more than 10,000 CEA studies.[4] Values of ℓ^* can also, of course, be estimated directly from ongoing clinical studies by assessing HRQoL of patients in the untreated state, for example.

Now we have the necessary data to determine R using some assumed values for the risk parameters, r^*_H, π^*_H, and τ^*_H. These values would come from separate studies using a discrete choice experiment or happiness economics as discussed in Chapter 8. The Taylor series estimate of the value of R, repeated here for convenience from Eq. (2.8), is:[5]

$$R = \left[1 + r^*_H \ell^* + \frac{1}{2} r^*_H \pi^*_H \ell^{*2} + \frac{1}{6} r^*_H \pi^*_H \tau^*_H + \dots \right] \qquad (9.3)$$

To complete our example, suppose that $\ell^* = 0.4$, a moderately severe health loss. If the affected person began in normal health ($H_0 = 1$) and the illness remained untreated, then HRQoL after the incidence of illness would become $H_{1S} = 0.6$.

Next, suppose that the estimated risk-preference parameters are $r^* = 0.7$, $\pi^* = 1.7$, and $\tau^* = 2.7$, indicating that utility in health is constant relative risk aversion (CRRA). From Table 2.1, $R = 1.43$. If non-CRRA utility is present, the specific parameters can be inserted into Eq. (9.3).[6] These specific parameters will have been estimated previously by other analysts and do not need to be measured for each HTA effort.

Again, reading from Table 2.1, for a more severe illness, if $\ell^* = 0.6$, then $R = 1.90$. For a highly severe illness where $\ell^* = 0.8$, then $R = 3.08$. These represent the marginal values of improving health from any specific treatment.

At this point, we again assure readers that the CRRA assumption is not required. The range of utility functions can be expanded substantially by employing the more general hyperbolic absolute risk aversion (HARA) utility function to estimate higher order risk parameters. Chapter 8 provides an extensive discussion of the HARA model, and we provide an example later in this chapter. Again, we remind the reader of the exact utility model as an alternative approach to the Taylor Series estimates (see Appendix 6.1).

Nonmarginal Changes in Treatment Efficacy

Here, we need to remind users of the consequences of nonmarginal changes in treatment efficacy, as discussed in Chapter 2. If an intervention shifts the level of health by a discrete (nonmarginal) change, then the average R value must be determined and then applied to the change in illness level. For example, from Table 2.2, if a patient begins with $\ell^* = 0.8$ (a severe health loss) which is improved by the medical intervention to $\ell^* = 0.3$, the gain is 0.5 on our HRQoL scale. From Table 2.2, if $r_H^* = 0.7$, then the cumulative R score is $(1.28 - 0.34) = 0.94$ for a 0.5 improvement on our HRQoL scale, which implies an average of $R = 1.88$. This calculation must be made for every nonmarginal improvement in health using either the numerical integration method discussed in Chapter 2 or the Taylor series alternative that we discuss in Chapter 11. This is unnecessary in standard CEA, where QALYs all have the same incremental value.

Incorporating the Elasticity of Utility of Health

Chapter 8 assesses in detail methods to calculate the elasticity of utility with respect to HRQoL, ω_H. Briefly summarizing here, the concepts of ω_H and r_H^* are closely related. In the simplest of models, in which utility has CRRA, $\omega_H + r_H^* = 1$, so when one knows either of these parameters, the other is also immediately apparent. As Chapter 8 elaborates, when we cannot assume that utility in HRQoL exhibits CRRA, we must also estimate the rate at which r_H^* and/or ω_H change as levels of health change. Using the highly general HARA utility function allows a smooth transition to the next step in the "assembly" of K_{GRACE}.

Combining Parameters to Estimate K_{GRACE}

Ignoring (for now) issues associated with permanent disability, we can now combine the three key elements of K_{GRACE} together to assess their net value, $K_{GRACE} = K\omega_H R$. To begin, it is useful to recall how K itself is determined.

In the British National original formulation of CEA, Garber and Phelps (1997) demonstrated that the optimal CEA threshold for WTP is given by $K = \dfrac{U(C)}{U'(C)}$, the ratio of utility to marginal utility of consumption. Phelps (2019a) elaborated on this measure, noting that one can define $K = \dfrac{C}{\omega_C}$, where ω_C is the elasticity of utility with respect to consumption of market goods and services. The lower the value of ω_C, the greater the WTP for improved health because the "cost" of foregone consumption is lower (as measured by ω_C). In the British National Health Service and elsewhere, some scholars view the opportunity cost as the foregone health from reducing other medical services to stay within a fixed budget constraint. Once K is determined, the GRACE methods apply, no matter whether K measures the opportunity cost as foregone consumption (Garber and Phelps, 1997; Phelps, 2019b) or foregone health (e.g., Claxton et al., 2015).

At this point, we are now in position to measure $\omega_H R$, the GRACE-related measure of WTP, and then express K_{GRACE} as a severity-specific multiplier for K. Combining K with these "K multipliers" completes the monetization of K_{GRACE}.

Monetary Values of K_{GRACE}

K_{GRACE} begins with K as the basis for valuation of health improvements, adding the two new elements, ω_H and R. Standard CEA requires that $\omega_H = 1$ and $R = 1$, meaning that the returns to improving health care are constant and that there is no adjustment for untreated disease severity. GRACE generalizes traditional CEA by allowing for diminishing returns for HRQoL ($\omega_H < 1$).

One fundamental conclusion emerges from the GRACE model: Traditional CEA overvalues health improvements for low-severity illnesses ($R \approx 1$) when there are diminishing returns to health improvements. The latter condition implies that $0 < \omega_H < 1$ (i.e., that the marginal utility of health is positive but declining). Then, necessarily, $\dfrac{\omega_H}{\omega_C} < \dfrac{1}{\omega_C}$. Since $R \approx 1$ for low-severity diseases, then $K\omega_H R < K$ for low-severity health conditions. The extent to which this affects overall valuation of health improvements depends on estimation of the actual values of ω_H and comparing them with known estimates of ω_C, and (of course) disease severity, since R grows nonlinearly as ℓ^* grows.

Table 9.1 MARGINAL K MULTIPLIERS FOR COMBINATIONS OF ω_H AND r_H^*

		ω_H	ℓ^*		
			0.4	0.6	0.8
$r_H^* + \omega_H = 1.200$	0.8	0.4	0.620	0.948	3.400
	0.4	0.8	0.992	1.220	2.120
$r_H^* + \omega_H = 1.100$	0.7	0.4	0.580	0.800	1.540
	0.4	0.7	0.861	1.036	1.512
$r_H^* + \omega_H = 1.000$	0.6	0.4	0.544	0.692	1.052
	0.4	0.6	0.738	0.858	1.140
$r_H^* + \omega_H = 0.900$	0.5	0.4	0.512	0.616	0.812
	0.4	0.5	0.610	0.705	0.880
$r_H^* + \omega_H = 0.800$	0.400	0.4	0.488	0.516	0.670

Notes: The leftmost column reports the respective value for the sum, $r_H^* + \omega_H$. For example, $r_H^* + \omega_H = 1.200$ represents the circumstance in which $r_H^* + \omega_H = 1.2$, and so on. $r_H^* + \omega_H = 1.00$ corresponds to CRRA utility. Values where $r_H^* + \omega_H > 1$ correspond to DRRA utility. Values where $r_H^* + \omega_H < 1$ correspond to IRRA utility. The values in the three right-hand columns represent K multipliers to convert K to K_{GRACE}.

Table 9.1 completes the monetization by providing multipliers that GRACE requires to adjust K. This table expands the potential range of values of ω_H and r_H^* by employing the HARA utility function, which allows $\omega_C + r_H^*$ to sum to values other than 1. In contrast, CRRA utility imposes the restriction that $\omega_C + r_H^* = 1$. Readers may wish to review the material in Chapter 8 regarding HARA utility to refresh their understanding of how using HARA utility allows use of the higher order terms in Eq. (2.8) for R.

The goal of Table 9.1 is to demonstrate how the K multiplier changes with different combinations of ω_C and r_H^*. In this table, values closer to 1.0 represent situations in which K_{GRACE} is closer to K. Values of the multiplier exceeding 1.0 indicate situations in which $K_{\text{GRACE}} > K$, and when the multiplier is less than 1.0, $K_{\text{GRACE}} < K$. The magnitude of the multiplier directly determines the relative change in the WTP for health improvement as the GRACE method is applied. Table 9.1 generalizes previous discussions in our presentation that were primarily limited to the situation in which utility was CRRA. Here, we demonstrate the consequences of relaxing that assumption through the use of the HARA utility function. Note that all of these are *marginal* values at specific values of ℓ^*.

To understand Table 9.1 fully, first focus on the gray-shaded rows, noting that in each of these rows, $\omega_H = 0.4$. In each companion unshaded row, the value of ω_H falls steadily as you work down the rows of the table. The cell entries in the final three columns describe the multiplier of K to convert it into the proper K_{GRACE} value. The middle row, $r_H^* + \omega_H = 1.000$, where utility is CRRA, denotes the transition between decreasing relative risk aversion (DRRA) and increasing relative risk aversion (IRRA). A total of 1.2 represents a significant level of DRRA, and a total of 0.8 represents a significant level of IRRA.

To elaborate on the content of Table 9.1, look at the top shaded row, where $r_H^* = 0.8$ and $\omega_H = 0.4$. The K multiplier rises from 0.62 (for $\ell^* = 0.4$) to 3.4 (for $\ell^* = 0.8$). This shows a very steep severity-of-illness gradient. The ratio of K multipliers from lowest to highest illness severity in this row is 5.5.

The same pattern holds as you successively work down, shaded row by shaded row, to lower values of r_H^*. However, as r_H^* falls with ω_H held constant at 0.4, the K multiplier becomes increasingly smaller.

Now look at the unshaded row in each pair of rows, descending from top to bottom of Table 9.1. In these cases, the values of ω_H and r_H^* have been reversed compared with their "companion" shaded rows, keeping the sum $r_H^* + \omega_H$ the same as its companion. In the top pair of rows $r_H^* + \omega_H = 1.200$, one can see that the valuation of the low-severity illness has increased from 0.62K to 0.99K, but the valuation for the highest severity illness has fallen from 3.4 to 2.12. In other words, the severity gradient flattens out as ω_H increases and r_H^* correspondingly shrinks. This same pattern is replicated in each successive pair of rows as one moves down the pairs in Table 9.1. The only difference is that as r_H^* declines (moving down the table), valuations at every level decline, and the severity gradient becomes increasingly flatter.

Two important lessons emerge from this analysis. First, the specific values of ω_H and r_H^* have considerable effect on valuations of medical interventions at different illness severity levels even when the total of $(r^* + \omega_H)$ remains constant. The severity gradients are steepest with high values of r_H^*. Similarly, the severity gradients flatten out as ω_H grows and r_H^* falls commensurately. At the extreme, when $\omega_H = 1$ and $r_H^* = 0$ (i.e., standard CEA), the severity gradient is completely flat because the valuation is $1 \times K$ at all illness severity levels.

The other observation from these results is that the K multiplier is less than 1 in many cases, particularly at lower severity levels (i.e., those with ℓ^* under 0.6). This phenomenon strongly interacts with the total value of $\omega_H + r_H^*$. When this sum is notably less than 1.0 (indicating IRRA), the K multiplier, $\omega_H R$, is almost universally less than 1. When the sum $(r^* + \omega_H)$ notably exceeds 1.0 (indicating significant DRRA), then overall valuation multipliers are regularly above 1, especially with higher values of ω_H. In this case, $K_{GRACE} > K$.

We do not know at this point which of these situations holds. The results will importantly depend on careful estimates of ω_H and r_H^* and their sum. This will broadly determine whether overall valuations of medical interventions will rise or fall with global implementation of GRACE.

This completes our discussion of how to assemble the K_{GRACE} value, except for introduction of the adjustment for permanent disability. The next section accomplishes that task.

INCORPORATING PERMANENT DISABILITY INTO K_{GRACE}^D

We consider disability as a permanent condition reducing people's health for which no treatment exists. If a treatment for such a disability becomes available, it can be treated just as any other acute illness in the GRACE framework. Disability has two distinct effects on our final measure of K_{GRACE}. First and by far the most important, it directly modifies K_{GRACE} to show that WTP for improvements in HRQoL rises steeply as the degree of permanent disability rises. We measure permanent disability, d^*, in the same way as we measure ℓ^*—that is, as a proportional loss in HRQoL. Therefore, the baseline health state for a person with a permanent disability is $H_{0d} = H_0(1 - d^*)$. The second effect is that disability decreases the baseline level of HRQoL, so when an acute illness afflicts a disabled person, the net effect leads to lower HRQoL than for an otherwise-similar nondisabled person. We discuss these two issues in order.

The Direct Effect of Preexisting Disability

Without disability included, $K_{\text{GRACE}} = K\omega_H R$. When permanent disability is included, Lakdawalla and Phelps (2022) show that ratio needs to be adjusted by the ratio $\dfrac{W(H_0)}{W(H_{0d})}$, the ratio of health-related utility in the "normal" state to utility in the permanently disabled state.[7] Furthermore, they show $\dfrac{W(H_0)}{W(H_{0d})} = \left[\dfrac{1}{1 - \psi d^*}\right] = D$, where $0 \leq \psi \leq 1$ and represents the consequences of diminishing returns to health on the way disability affects utility of health. If the exact utility version of GRACE is used, the ratio of utilities can be directly estimated, of course. Then:

$$K_{\text{GRACE}}^D = KD\omega_H R \tag{9.4}$$

If $d^* = 0$, K_{GRACE} is unaffected by disability, but if $d^* > 0$, K_{GRACE} rises. The effect can be quite large for severe disabilities. For example, if $\psi d^* = 0.5$, K_{GRACE} doubles. The adjustment ψd^* uses the Taylor series expansion of the ratio of the two utilities, $\dfrac{W(H_{0d})}{W(H_0)}$:

$$\psi d^* = \omega_H d^*\left[1 + \left(\frac{1}{2}\right)r_H^* d^* + \left(\frac{1}{6}\right)\pi_H^* r_H^* d^{*2} + \left(\frac{1}{24}\right)\tau_H^* \pi_H^* r_H^* d^{*3} + \ldots\right] \tag{9.5}$$

Table 9.2 shows examples of how disability and diminishing returns interact. In these examples, we continue to use CRRA utility, and within that

Table 9.2 DISABILITY ADJUSTMENT $= D = \dfrac{1}{1 - \psi d^*}$

r^*	Disability Severity (d^*)									
	0	0.1	0.2	0.3	0.4	0.5	0.6	0.7	0.8	0.9
0	1	1.10	1.25	1.43	1.67	2.00	2.50	3.33	5.00	10.00
0.1	1	1.1	1.22	1.38	1.58	1.87	2.28	3.00	4.26	7.94
0.3	1	1.08	1.17	1.28	1.42	1.62	1.90	2.32	3.08	5.01
0.5	1	1.06	1.13	1.20	1.30	1.41	1.58	1.82	2.24	3.16
0.7	1	1.03	1.07	1.13	1.17	1.23	1.32	1.44	1.62	1.99
0.9	1	1.01	1.02	1.04	1.05	1.07	1.10	1.13	1.17	1.25

structure, we calculate values of $D = \left[\dfrac{1}{1 - \psi d^*} \right]$ for different combinations of r_H^* and d^*. In Table 9.2, remember that CRRA implies $r_H^* + \omega_H = 1$, so as r_H^* rises, ω_H commensurately falls in the calculation of ψ.[8]

In Table 9.2, the leftmost columns show that for all levels of r_H^*, the adjustment is small for small values of d^*, and that adjustment value declines to near 1.0 as r_H^* approaches 1.0 (meaning that ω_H approaches 0). The adjustment rises steadily (columns further and further to the right) as d^* rises, the effect being greatest when r_H^* is smaller and hence ω_H is larger.

Note that if in our model we were to set $r_H^* = 0$ and at the same time to relax the standard CEA modeling assumption that $H_0 = 1$, then the adjustment factor (where $\psi = 1$) is $\dfrac{1}{1 - d^*}$. This leads to adjustment factors of 1.11 for $d^* = 0.1$, 2.0 for $d^* = 0.5$, and, up to 10 for $d^* = 0.9$. In this case, note also that $R = 1$ when $r_H^* = 0$.

Combining Acute Illness and Permanent Disability in R

The second effect of disability arises indirectly in the calculation of the severity parameter R. For any given degree of severity of an acute illness,

ℓ^*, the presence of a preexisting permanent disability, d^*, worsens the final untreated health status.

No clearly agreed upon methods exist to combine ℓ^* and d^*. The proper method would elicit HRQoL values for people with all potential combinations of permanent disability directly, a process that would presumably yield results where $0 \le H < 1$. This process remains infeasible at this point, and probably "forever," because the number of potential respondents could be very small for combinations of rare disease and rare permanent disability.[9]

To deal with this problem in real-world CEA assessments, analysts have commonly turned to two approaches—additive and multiplicative modeling. In the additive model, $H = H_0(1 - \ell^* - d^*)$. This has the unfortunate consequence that it can lead to values of $H < 0$ on a scale where "0" is the "worst imaginable health status" or something comparable.

The alternative uses a multiplicative model, where $H = H_0(1 - \ell^*)(1 - d^*)$, which always has values of $H > 0$ but says that disabled people lose less health-related HRQoL from acute illness than nondisabled people. Note that the difference is small unless $\ell^* d^*$ is large since $(1 - \ell^*)(1 - d^*) = (1 - \ell^* - d^* + d^* \ell^*)$. We do not intend to (nor need we) resolve this dispute, noting that the proper approach would determine HRQoL levels empirically from people with the combined illness and permanent disability. Our model simply assumes that d^* has properly been combined with ℓ^*. This combined value is the proper level of illness severity to use in computing the severity of illness ratio R.

The Marginal Rate of Substitution Parameter ρ

The parameter ρ measures the ratio of expected utility of health for sick-but-treated patients relative to expected utility in perfect health, so $\rho = \dfrac{E(W(H_{1T}))}{W(H_0)}$. In general, $\rho < 1$ unless there is no disability and the treatment provides a perfect cure of the illness in question:

$$\rho = 1 - \omega_H t^* \left[1 + \frac{1}{2} r_H^* t^* + \frac{1}{6} r_H^* \pi_H^* t^{*2} + \frac{1}{24} r_H^* \pi_H^* \tau_H^* t^{*3} + \ldots \right] \quad (9.6)$$

Obviously, if treatments are 100% effective and there is no disability, then $\rho = 1$.

If Eq. (9.6) looks eerily familiar, that is because ρ has the identical mathematical structure as that of the adjustment for permanent disability, ψd^*, as shown in Eq. (9.5), except that t^* is substituted for d^*. Both are calculating the Taylor series expansion for the ratio of two expected utility values, so it should come as no surprise that they have similar structure.

The relevant calculations to compute ρ are simply sums of products, a task that is easily performed, for example, in any standard spreadsheet software. As an example of the computation of ρ, assume that the utility of health is CRRA with $r_H^* = 0.5$, so $\omega_H = 0.5$, $\pi_H^* = 1.5$, and $\tau_H^* = 2.5$, and so on.[10] Now, if $t^* = 0.2$ (e.g., an illness loss of $\ell^* = 0.6$ and a mean treatment benefit of $\mu_B = 0.4$), then the term in square braces in Eq. (9.6) equals 1.056 and $\rho = 0.894$, a relatively small loss in the expected utility of HRQoL compared with $W(H_0)$.

Using the same risk-parameter values as before, with a permanent disability level of $d^* = 0.4$, the term in square braces in Eq. (9.6) equals 1.12 and $\rho = 0.775$. Continuing the example, if $d^* = 0.6$, ρ falls to 0.63. At a very severe disability of $d^* = 0.8$, $\rho = 0.447$. Clearly, the MRS can be very sensitive to the extent of permanent disability.

As is also obvious at this point, ρ will differ for otherwise-identical people with and without permanent disabilities. For any given values of ℓ^*, the untreated illness loss, and the treatment benefit B, a person with $d^* > 0$ will have a lower treated outcome, and hence a lower value of t^*.

The other (equivalent) interpretation of this, of course, is that disabled people are more willing to trade LE to gain HRQoL. This makes perfect intuitive sense. People who have a lower HRQoL from a disability gain greater utility for any given increase in HRQoL because of diminishing returns to H.

At this point, it is also worth noting the consequences of assuming (as does standard CEA) that there are no declining returns to HRQoL, so that $\omega_H = 1$, $R = 1$, and r_H^*, and all higher order risk terms equal 0. Then $\rho = 1 - t^*$ and the MRS becomes $\delta = H_0(1 - t^*)$. This is exactly the MRS used in traditional CEA models, in which the MRS equals H_{1T}, the period 1 health level after treatment.

The Outcome Uncertainty Multiplier, ε

The GRACE model requires one further adjustment to traditional CEA to properly incorporate measures of health improvements. Remember that the acronym GRACE includes the words "risk-adjusted." To accomplish the appropriate risk adjustment, we must first adjust the average health improvement, μ_B, by incorporating relevant measures of the variability of health outcomes in T and C, summarized by changes in variances, skewness, and (where available) kurtosis of the distribution of health outcomes. This is the certainty equivalent multiplier ε, which adjusts for the risk associated with variable treatment outcomes. If T and C have identical risk profiles, then $\varepsilon = 1$, but that value can rise or fall depending on the risk profiles of T and C and the degrees of risk aversion, r_H^*, and related risk parameters.

The value ε adjusts mean improvements in HRQoL (when comparing two therapies, T and C) to take account of uncertain treatment outcomes and the ways which that uncertainty is valued by consumers who are risk averse in HRQoL. For typical risk preferences, less variance in outcomes is often desirable, but positive skewness (increasing the chances of a wonderful outcome) is also desirable.[11] The formula for ε [repeating Eq. (4.1) here] is[12]

$$
\varepsilon \approx 1 + \left\{ \frac{\mu_H}{\mu_B} \right\} \left[\begin{array}{c} -\dfrac{1}{2} r_H^* \left(\dfrac{1}{\mu_H} \right)^2 \Delta\sigma_H^2 + \dfrac{1}{6} \pi_H^* r_H^* \left(\dfrac{1}{\mu_H} \right)^3 \Delta[\gamma_1 \sigma_H^3] \\[2ex] -\dfrac{1}{24} \tau_H^* \pi_H^* r_H^* \left(\dfrac{1}{\mu_H} \right)^2 \Delta[\gamma_2 \sigma_H^4]\dots \end{array} \right] \tag{9.7}
$$

In Eq. (9.7), the risk-preference parameters should be evaluated at a health level of $H = H_0(1 - \ell^*)$.

The ratio $\left\{ \dfrac{\mu_H}{\mu_B} \right\}$ importantly affects the final value. If μ_B is relatively large, the "risk" terms have less importance in determining total value in the total value of a medical intervention expression. Similarly, the average HRQoL value of an untreated sick person, μ_H, also affects the outcome. The "risk components" have less importance to sicker people (who have a low value of μ_H), other things equal.

The ε multiplier applies to the mean benefit, μ_B. If $\varepsilon = 1$, the result from GRACE in terms of equivalent HRQoL changes is the same as with traditional CEA. In other words, a one-unit gain in average (stochastic) HRQoL is just as valuable as a one-unit gain in actual HRQoL. If $\varepsilon > 1$, then the total HRQoL gain is worth more than traditional CEA assumes, and conversely if $\varepsilon < 1$. Recall that standard CEA assumes that r_H^* and all higher risk-preference terms equal 0, so $\varepsilon = 1$.

Looking at Eq. (9.7), the statistical components come from clinical studies, which provide the values for $\Delta\sigma_H^2$, $[\gamma_1\sigma_H^3]$, $\Delta[\gamma_2\sigma_H^4]$, etc. All that these new data require are simple extra calculations from the raw data that every clinical study would normally accumulate.

Assembling the estimate for ε simply requires following Eq. (9.7) closely. The first step measures the variances of T and C, and then takes their difference. That difference is then normalized by $\left(\dfrac{1}{\mu_H} \right)^2$ to make it scale-free. Then the same is done for skewness measures (normalizing by $\left(\dfrac{1}{\mu_H} \right)^3$), and so forth. Then these normalized differences are weighted by the Taylor series multipliers, $\dfrac{1}{2}r_H^*$, $\dfrac{1}{6}r_H^*\pi_H^*$, etc., and then added up. That gives the value for ε.

SUMMARY

Combining the elements of GRACE into a complete measure of the value of medical interventions requires two types of new data. The first of these are the risk-preference parameters that define people's attitudes toward diminishing returns to health and uncertain treatment outcomes. In this chapter, we have assumed that such parameters are "known" to the analyst, and we have explored the consequences of having different values emerge from the studies estimating these parameters. In general, these are "done-once" parameters that need not be repeated in each analysis of each new medical technology.

The second set of parameters must be estimated in every HTA. Just as with standard CEA models, GRACE requires differences in mean outcomes of T and C for HRQoL and LE (defined in our model respectively as μ_B and μ_P). In addition, GRACE requires information about the uncertainty of treatment outcomes, including variances, skewness, and, if possible, kurtosis of the distributions of health outcomes in T and C.

The key differences between GRACE and the standard CEA model can be illuminated well in the single-period model. The shift from that analysis to a multiperiod model with stationary parameters is relatively straightforward. The full multiperiod model is then shown to be essentially the same as the single-period model with the exception that the key parameters in the model all must be estimated on a period-by-period basis. After that, estimating a full multiperiod model essentially involves bookkeeping to keep track of the period-by-period values and adding them up over time. As discussed in Chapter 6, standard clinical trials and the majority of standard cost-effectiveness models will provide proper estimates of untreated average survival probability, p_n^U, treated average survival probability, p_n^T, and their difference, the average gain in LE, $\mu_{P_n} = p_n^T - p_n^U$, commonly measured with techniques such as Kaplan–Meier estimators (Kaplan and Meier, 1958).

Permanent disability affects the GRACE model in three ways. GRACE unambiguously increases the valuation of improvements in HRQoL as disability increases. The first effect arises directly through the disability factor D. The second arises through the increase in illness severity as acute illness and disability effects are combined.

This proves that when it comes to valuing the third effect focuses on valuation of increases in LE. Because diminishing returns affect the marginal rate of substitution between LE and HRQoL, the GRACE model shows that as disability increases, the MRS factor, δ, decreases as disability severity increases. Therefore, the value of increases in LE becomes an issue that can only be resolved empirically on a case-by-case basis. The first two effects compete with the third in determining the final outcome. The disability-adjustment factor, D, and illness severity, R, increase the value of LE increases, whereas the exchange rate between HRQoL and LE, δ, decreases it. Chapter 5 provides some guidance on when we can ensure that the value of LE increases as disability increases.

The similarity in structure between the estimates for the parameters d^* and t^* makes another point clear: The adjustment for disability, D, and ρH_0 are inverses of each other when $d^* = t^*$. This means that when $d^* = t^*$, the product $\rho D = 1$. This is important in assessing the net effect of GRACE calculations on the value of treating persons with permanent disabilities. When $\rho D = 1$, the net value of extending LE is simply $K\mu_p$, which is the same as for a nondisabled person. If a treatment has *any* beneficial effect to improve health above d^*, then $t^* < d^*$ and $\rho D > 1$. This proves that when it comes to valuing any intervention that improves a permanent disability, GRACE unambiguously values LE gains for disabled people as greater than for equivalent LE gains for otherwise similar non-disabled people. This occurs in addition to the previously discussed notion that GRACE unambiguously values gains in HRQoL as greater for disabled than for otherwise similar non-disabled people. Thus, in this case, the TVMI in GRACE assures greater value for any treatment improving disabilities that does not involve an acute illness.

Transition Issues

Intelligence is the ability to adapt to change.

—Stephen Hawking

How do we get from "here" to "there" in standard health technology assessment (HTA) practices? This chapter discusses some of the transition issues that could arise when health plans shift from status quo HTA to generalized risk-adjusted cost-effectiveness (GRACE) model–based methods. We organize this around two main issues.

The first concerns how to implement severity-based valuations (the parameter R in the GRACE model). The second arises from analyses presented in Chapter 7, which strongly suggests that the optimal threshold, K, and therefore also K_{GRACE}, varies positively with income. This raises the question of how, or even whether, to implement HTA that allows thresholds to vary with income. This is addressed later in the chapter. We explore these two issues in turn.

IMPLEMENTING SEVERITY ADJUSTMENTS

GRACE clarifies that consumers with declining marginal utility from health (and, equivalently, risk averse over health gains) are made better off if their insurance plans adjust the willingness to pay (WTP) threshold to account for illness severity. This is not merely a conceptual exercise.

Valuing Health. Charles E. Phelps and Darius N. Lakdawalla, Oxford University Press. © Oxford University Press 2024. DOI: 10.1093/oso/9780197686287.003.0010

Several health plans throughout the world (most notably, those in Europe) have already incorporated specific severity adjustments into their formal cost-effectiveness thresholds. The value of doing this—if properly done— follows directly from the analysis in Chapter 2, and we consider it vital. However, the literature has not yet agreed upon a method for assessing severity of illness in these situations, nor has it agreed upon the best ways to adjust WTP for illness severity, once the latter is identified and measured.

Chapter 12 provides some background information about alternative ways to measure value that do not rely directly on consumer preferences. These methods, called "extra welfarism," contrast with standard cost-effectiveness analysis (CEA) and GRACE methods, which rely wholly on consumer preferences as measures of value. Chapter 12 then summarizes and evaluates three ad hoc severity adjustments that some European nations now use. These do not use value measures that rely on consumer preferences; rather, they use those that rely on various definitions of "equity" to support their various adjustment measures. In this chapter, we continue to rely on consumer preferences, as developed in GRACE, as the proper measure of value.

GRACE provides a theory-based method for measuring illness severity (using existing tools and methods, all of which will improve over time). Still needed for GRACE are estimates of the way the utility of health behaves (our ω_H) as the level of health changes. Standard CEA assumes (incorrectly, we believe) that $\omega_H = 1$.

The extent to which WTP rises with severity depends significantly on these yet-unmeasured risk-preference values (ω_H, r_H^* and higher order risk-preference terms). Sensitivity analyses in Chapter 11 demonstrate the importance of these parameters in determining the best severity-adjustment profile. Without such estimates in hand, we cannot recommend specific severity profiles, but we believe that the GRACE method provides a clear pathway to establishing tractable, valid, and rigorous severity adjustments to WTP thresholds, once the relevant preference parameters are estimated.

Although we have previously referenced several studies demonstrating people's WTP more for losses to people with highly severe illnesses, a

Japanese study provides a good context setting for what follows. Shiroiwa et al. (2013) gathered data from 2,400 respondents from an online panel, presenting to each respondent questionnaires concerning one of 16 health status situations, with severity calibrated by EQ-5D methods. By way of background, the authors state that Japanese yen (JPY) 5 to 6 million per quality-adjusted life year (QALY; approximately $60,000 to $75,00) is a standard "reference value" in Japan. In hypothetical illness situations, respondents were asked if they wanted to purchase treatment for the disorder, and WTP estimates were inferred accordingly. The results indicate that WTP per QALY ranged from approximately JPY 2 million per QALY for low-severity illnesses to JPY 8 million for the highest severity situations, with the slope of approximately JPY 1 million per 0.1 QALY gain.

These results are wholly consistent with the methods developed in GRACE, and in some sense they provide a backdoor estimate to the parameter values, which could be inferred by mapping these WTP results to multipliers shown in Table 2.1. We draw this conclusion by comparing the ratio of multiplier for low- and high-severity diseases. In Shiroiwa et al.'s (2013) data, the ratio of WTP for high severity to low severity is approximately 4.0. This is roughly consistent with values in Table 2.1 of $r_H^* = 0.6$, where the multipliers for the two highest illness severity categories are 3.62 and 5.01. This 4X multiplier also appears in other severity adjustments that Chapter 12 discusses. We note, however, that this is not designed to be a rigorous measure of relative risk aversion in health but, rather, an illustrative piece of evidence documenting the qualitative theoretical predictions of the GRACE model for WTP.

Single-Payer Health Systems

Any single-payer health system (e.g., the British National Health System [BNHS]) could implement severity-adjusted value systems to support decisions about when to include or exclude treatments from the list of covered services and biopharmaceutical products from their "formulary." The same would be true for any single-payer universal health insurance plan, such as Canada's Medicare system or the U.S. Medicare system for persons aged 65 years and other persons with permanent disabilities. The transition to GRACE is simply an organizational decision (unless, of course, such changes are prohibited by law).

Wider implementation of severity-based systems could involve a shift in payments to providers, which is an issue when the single-payer system operates wholly as an insurance plan, such as Canada's Medicare system. This occurs when systems shift from measuring value to actual payment levels for providers. In the short term, such a shift could alter the relative earnings of various medical providers, causing longer term shifts in human resources distribution. This might include, for example, shifts in primary care provision from physicians to nurse practitioners, changes in post-graduate medical education (residencies and fellowships), and even inter-national migration of providers. These are not immediate consequences of using GRACE or other methods of value but, rather, arise when provider payments become linked to those value measures.

Competitive Markets

In the United States (with which we have the greatest familiarity) and else-where, health insurance is not provided by a single governmental payer but, rather, by competing insurance organizations, some of which (e.g., health maintenance organizations) might provide health care directly, and others might steer patients to "preferred providers" that have agreed to specific reimbursement levels as compensation for their services.

Pauly (2017) has envisioned how a competitive marketplace might function with different health plans offering different CEA thresholds to consumers who would choose the threshold most compatible with their own preferences (and income). It is but a small step from Pauly's conceptu-alization of health plans offering different thresholds to a system including plans offering GRACE-like severity gradients in decision thresholds.

To our understanding, no health plans formally use CEA in the United States. However, there is apparently extensive informal use of CEA in the formulary setting among health plans and even in the recommendations of the committee that recommends vaccine use to the Centers for Disease Control and Prevention.

We can envision a competitive insurance market where robust competition exists on generosity of insurance plans. One obvious dimension is the "scope of benefits" list of covered services, a list that applies to all enrollees. Formularies serve the same function for biopharmaceutical products, and most insurance plans specifically exclude coverage of experimental treatments. The other dimension involves choices on the extensive and intensive margins for use of approved therapies. This issue harkens back to Chapter 1, wherein we discussed the importance of these "margins" in determining cost-effectiveness of various medical interventions.

Many U.S. health plans manage these decisions through "prior authorization" processes designed to stop or to discourage the expanded use of valid medical care interventions along the intensive margins (e.g., no more than one "general physical exam a year" or no more than two dental "prophylaxis" visits per year) or the extensive margin (e.g., age limits on coverage of various preventive interventions and diagnostic tests such as colonoscopy).[1] Thus, the operational strategies of health plans in the United States currently may carry out many of the activities that formal CEA might strengthen. We argue, of course, that these would be accomplished more accurately (in reflecting patient preferences) if the GRACE model of valuation was the centerpiece of these choices.

Implementation of major shifts toward severity adjustment in single-payer systems requires a decision about what adjustment process to use, and possibly budget reallocations to support necessary operational changes. In private insurance plans in the United States, such a decision would almost certainly require both administrative support and approval from the organization's governing board. The major issue, when health insurance markets are competitive, is consumer acceptance of such a plan and the possibility of inducing shifts both in patient enrollment and, where appropriate, approved panels of health care providers.

A possible "selection bias" issue looms large here (Rothschild and Stiglitz, 1976). Individual plans implementing a severity-based system for measuring value would presumably shift resources toward treating more severely ill patients and away from milder cases. This could induce the healthiest patients to seek other coverage and attract sicker patients who had previously enrolled in other plans. Evaluation of how such market equilibria would emerge is a fruitful topic of further study.

Guidance from GRACE

Existing European approaches to incorporating severity of illness raise several fundamental questions, all of which are discussed extensively in Phelps and Lakdawalla (2023). Three of the most basic questions are whether health loss measurements should be absolute or proportional and, if the latter, "proportional to what?" The second question, closely related, asks how age and remaining life expectancy (LE) should matter. The third question asks whether health losses in the past should matter, that is, methods that incorporate "health loss from birth," sometimes called the "fair innings" approach, in the measure of value of improving health. Chapter 12 discusses these approaches in greater detail from the perspective of "social welfare" measurements that aggregate values for individual members of the society. We ignore these European measures at this point because they rely on ad hoc equity arguments rather than on economic models of consumer preferences.

GRACE answers these questions from the viewpoint of a rational, risk-averse, "representative" individual with diminishing returns to HRQoL. From that perspective, GRACE (and standard CEA) is clear on the third of these issues: It is forward-looking and does not incorporate past health status, except insofar as it informs future health status.[2] The fair innings approach is inconsistent with GRACE methodology and, indeed, the entire body of centuries of economic analysis that is forward-looking.

Regarding the second question, both GRACE and standard CEA add up potential future benefits (discounted, in both cases) but with a finite remaining LE incorporated into the analysis. Thus, for example, preventing the death or improving the HRQoL of an 80-year-old provides less value in total than achieving the same for a 60-year-old. The formalization of this appears in Chapter 6, wherein the GRACE version of multiperiod valuation is presented. In Eq. 6.1, net monetary benefit of an intervention is the sum from $n = 1$ to N of health gains (net of costs). In normal practice, N would equal the periods of remaining LE for the person receiving the health gain.

Again, remember that this conclusion derives from the preferences of a single representative individual who is rational and risk averse. The reason for this outcome goes back to the most fundamental idea of standard CEA and GRACE: The opportunity cost of improved health is current consumption, so the fewer the number of remaining years of health gains that an intervention promises, the less our "rational representative consumer" would be willing to pay in terms of foregone consumption to receive such an intervention. Any bequest motives could further strenghten this conclusion.

Chapter 12 discusses in detail the problems that arise when one evaluates the existing European severity adjustment methods compared with GRACE. This is, of course, somewhat of an apples–oranges issue because GRACE rests on the premise of forward-looking behavior by a rational utility maximizer, whereas the European systems rest at least in part on ethical evaluations of fairness. However, we think it useful to assess how these currently embraced systems compare to GRACE.

INCOME-RELATED THRESHOLDS

Chapter 7, through a series of different approaches, shows that the optimal decision threshold for HTA, whether using standard CEA or GRACE, likely varies positively with income. A series of international comparisons makes this very evident at the national level, suggesting that K rises more rapidly than income so that improved health is a "luxury good" in the usual economic classification (i.e., income elasticity exceeds 1.0). The structural model approach (Phelps, 2017; Phelps and Cinatl, 2021) demonstrates the same phenomenon with two quite different utility functions used in the modeling. In this section, we address issues associated with implementing CEA thresholds that incorporate positive income gradients.

Competitive Markets

In a competitive market system such as Pauly (2017) envisioned, competition among plans provides a direct method for those with higher WTP to obtain their desired coverage. Indeed, even a single insurer might offer increasing coverage packages, priced to account for the increased costs associated with greater treatment availability. In current U.S. plans, this is managed not through a formal use of announced CEA thresholds but, rather, through pharmaceutical formulary composition (and tier assignment for patient co-payments), general coverage decisions, and (with regard to intensive and extensive margins determining who is eligible for various treatments) prior authorization rules and processes.

We can readily envision vigorous competition on this dimension of insurance coverage once wider use of CEA (and GRACE) emerges. To date in the United States, the only announced formal use of CEA thresholds was the CVS Pharmacy plan that limits access to drugs with incremental cost-effectiveness ratios under $100,000. However, CEA analyses by the Institute for Clinical and Economic Review in the United States are now widely cited.[3] Their work appears to have important leverage in insurance plans' decision-making about incorporating new treatments.

Single-Payer Health Plans

Universal coverage health plans exist in many forms throughout the world, in almost all cases with some sort of centralized government entity involved in either operating the health system or providing health insurance to the entire population. In the United States, the Medicare system for persons older than age 65 years and permanently disabled persons is such a system. Canada's Medicare system is similar, except that it covers the entire population. These systems differ on one important dimension: The U.S. Medicare system allows individuals to purchase supplemental insurance to reduce out-of-pocket payments on covered services.[4] Canada forbids such supplementation.

Allowing supplementation provides an outlet for consumers who desire more extensive coverage than the basic plan of a universal insurance system. Whenever optimal scope of benefits varies with income, allowing supplemental insurance increases the well-being of individuals who would otherwise live within the confines of the universal plan's single value.

Counterarguments in favor of banning supplementation include the notions that social cohesion is enhanced (1) by the "everybody is in the same lifeboat" situation and (2) by the more cynical view that banning supplementation will lead political decision-makers to pick more generous plans that meet their own personal preferences for plans that apply universally to entire populations (including the decision-making politicians).

Choosing a Single Value for a Universal Plan

This leads us to a brief discussion of how nations or states might choose a single threshold that applies to the entire population. Several models of political decision-making emerge that suggest how this might be done.

MEDIAN VOTER MODELS

Simple voting models provide simple answers to this question. If the affected population were to vote on a single threshold wherein each voter specified their most preferred value, then the optimal value for the median voter would prevail—a well-understood axiom of social choice theory. Given the skewed income distribution that prevails in almost all democracies, the median voter would have a lower income than the per capita gross domestic product (GDP) value. Yet almost all discussions of optimal thresholds in political arenas throughout the world focus on the optimal threshold being some multiplier of per capita GDP, a concept that was introduced formally by World Health Organization discussions of optimal thresholds. This at least implies that modes of thinking differ from "median voter" models when nations set specific WTP thresholds. With the reasonable premise that the optimal threshold rises with income (as most of the data and modeling suggest), median voting models would almost certainly lead to a single threshold value that was smaller than the optimum, perhaps by a significant amount.

LEGISLATIVE CHOICE

Only on few occasions are complex issues put directly to voters, and then (typically) in a simple yes/no format. The Brexit vote, although only advisory to the UK Parliament, provides a recent example involving a yes/no choice ("stay" or "leave"). Only on rare occasions do citizens vote on "a number" as would be required to have a vote-based value for K. More commonly, such choices are made by legislative bodies where the outcome may be determined at least in part by the composition and voting preferences of committees and subcommittees of the formal legislative body. These discussion seldom, if ever, focus on the specific value of K but, rather, on budgets for the health care system. This in turn produces the "shadow value" of K, the implicit cost-effectiveness threshold.

This can lead to potentially contradictory policies. For example, in Britain, the Department of the Treasury recommends use of £60,000 per QALY for valuing a life year, whereas the National Institute for Health and Care Excellence operates with an announced threshold of £30,000. However, the budget provided by the Treasury to the National Health Service leads to a shadow price of approximately £13,000 per QALY (Claxton et al., 2015).

Analyzing how such legislative actions are determined lies far beyond the scope of this book, and we tend to rely on the notion that "like sausage, you don't want to know very much about how such decisions are made."

MODELS FROM WELFARE ECONOMICS

The field of welfare economics assesses how to combine the utilities (levels of happiness) of individual members of a society into a societal measure by somehow aggregating the individual utilities. Some of these shed light on the meaning of choices of particular thresholds or (more particularly) the implications of choosing thresholds that do or do not vary with illness severity and disability. Chapter 12 discusses these approaches in more detail.

SUMMARY

Severity-Based Valuations

GRACE makes clear (from the viewpoint of a rational, expected utility-maximizing person who is risk averse in HRQoL) that proper valuation of HRQoL-based health improvements includes a continuous severity gradient, wherein more severe illnesses have higher value for the same amount of improvement in HRQoL than lower severity illnesses. GRACE also makes clear that it is not just the "starting point" that matters (i.e., the untreated illness severity, ℓ^*) but also the extent of recovery (t^*). The average valuation across the range of recovery is necessary to properly reflect a "representative consumer's" preferences. Implementations of severity-based thresholds in Europe have departed from these principles and pursued ad hoc approaches.

Income-Related Thresholds

COMPETITIVE MARKETS

Implementing income-related thresholds requires little other than allowing markets to work. In competitive insurance markets, such as in the United States, there is evidence that competition can emerge on issues closely related to cost-effectiveness thresholds. A good example emerges from the market for Medicare Advantage (Part C) insurance in Medicare. In that plan, eligibility for standard Medicare Part A (which is mandatory) and Part B (which is voluntary, but enrollees, by statute, pay only one-fourth of the expected cost) can be converted into what amounts to a voucher to purchase private insurance—the Medicare Advantage program.

Numerous insurance companies compete in this marketplace. They have at least three ways in which they can modify their offerings that are quite similar to altering a cost-effectiveness threshold. The first comes with the scope of benefits—the list of covered services. Medicare Advantage plans are free to expand their plans as long as they cover every service that "traditional" Medicare covers. This amounts to changes in coverage "on the extensive margin," to use the language of the discussion in Chapter 1.

They can also alter the stringency with which they approve or deny services, primarily through processes such as "prior authorization," wherein providers must gain approval of the insurance plan before undertaking some specified procedures. Plans gain reputations about their generosity or stringency on this dimension of coverage. It controls utilitization "on the intensive margin" in the language of Chapter 1.

Medicare Advantage plans also combine coverage for hospitalization and ambulatory care (Medicare Part A and Part B services) with Part D coverage of prescription drugs. The structure of these plans, including, for example, formulary inclusion or exclusion and "pricing tier" decisions about co-payments for prescription drugs, offers yet another dimension of competition among such plans that allows expansion on both intensive and extensive margins for prescription drugs.

It is but a small step to envision competition among insurance plans using a formal cost-effectiveness threshold once such systems come into wider use. From there, a simple step is plans offering differing thresholds, allowing people to satisfy their wishes for higher thresholds if they wish (and can afford it) to acquire more-generous plans than "basic" plans offer.

CENTRALIZED HEALTH SYSTEMS

In centralized health care systems such as are more common in Europe, augmentation of cost-effectiveness thresholds is most easily viewed as a public policy decision about whether insurance supplementation of basic plan offerings is permitted. In the United Kingdom, for example, individuals can purchase care from so-called Harley Street providers outside of the basic BNHS system, and insurance to cover such service has also emerged.

In contrast, Canada forbids supplementation of its universal Medicare plan. However, bypassing those restrictions, a considerable (but as yet unmeasured) amount of medical care for Canadian citizens takes place across the border in the United States. To maintain their Canadian coverage, people must reside in Canada for at least 153 days per year. Those who travel to the United States for medical care can buy "travelers' insurance" that covers U.S. medical care. These people are called "snowbird" travelers, but they can buy what amounts to health insurance by purchasing travelers' insurance. A robust market for "cross-border health insurance" advisors in Canada helps facilitate these decisions.

In summary, implementing income-based thresholds in centralized systems essentially comes down to a single decision about allowing or forbidding supplemental insurance. If such coverage is allowed, we envision that markets will do what they do best—meet the demands of potential customers. In those cases, increases in individuals' thresholds by income (or for whatever desired reason) should occur naturally. If such plans are forbidden, individuals will be denied the opportunity to fulfill their own preferences.

Consequences for Health Plans

Life is a series of natural and spontaneous changes.
Don't resist them; that only creates sorrow. Let reality be reality.
Let things flow naturally forward in whatever way they like.

—Lao Tzu

INTRODUCTION

Chapter 10 discussed questions involving implementation of the generalized risk-adjusted cost-effectiveness (GRACE) model–based valuation methods both in single-system settings and in competitive markets such as in the United States. This chapter addresses the related question, "So what?" How much does it matter whether standard cost-effectiveness analysis (CEA) or GRACE are used, and in what ways? And if "things change," what are the consequences for health plans and organizations? This chapter addresses these issues.

In part, this chapter is motivated by numerous questions that we have received during presentations of GRACE and, in some cases, extensive concern about the consequences for health plans if they adopt GRACE methods instead of standard CEA. Most of these issues focus on the effects of the multiplier R in the formula for K_{GRACE} with a concern that costs of providing care will rise precipitously because R exceeds 1.0, often by a considerable degree. This concern overlooks two issues. The first is the offsetting

Valuing Health. Charles E. Phelps and Darius N. Lakdawalla, Oxford University Press. © Oxford University Press 2024.
DOI: 10.1093/oso/9780197686287.003.0011

effect of introducing declining marginal utility of health, expressed as ω_H in the full measure of K_{GRACE}. From economic theory, $0 < \omega_H < 1$, which means that this factor lower valuations, offsetting increases that might arise from R.

However, another issue looms even larger: GRACE is not a price-setting method but, rather, a value-measuring method. We turn to this issue next.

VALUE VERSUS PRICING

We begin with what may seem obvious but remains important to reiterate: GRACE is not a price-setting method. It is a method to measure the value that a single, expected-utility-maximizing representative individual would place on any medical intervention. There are now many calls for "value-based pricing" in health care, particularly with regard to biopharmaceutical and medical device innovations (e.g., Danzon et al., 2015). However, these approaches do not necessarily imply that maximum willingness to pay (WTP) measures are the appropriate price; they merely call for a link between price and the value perceived by consumers.

K_{GRACE}, just as with the cost-effectiveness threshold K, is a maximum WTP. For "lumpy" interventions that cannot be adjusted continuously along an extensive or intensive margin (see discussion in Chapter 1), "value" has a different meaning. Many health care interventions have incremental cost-effectiveness ratios (ICERs) that fall well below announced WTP thresholds. This can occur because of lumpiness in the intervention's structure or because of incomplete expansion of use of "low-ICER interventions" on the extensive or intensive margins. If an intervention (at current levels of use) has an ICER less than the threshold, then expanding its use (if the technology allows this) up to the point where the ICER equals the threshold will improve consumers' well-being. If the technology is lumpy so that expansions on the extensive or intensive margins are impossible, then, for any fixed quantity, when price falls below maximum WTP, some surplus accrues to consumers. Consumer surplus adds up the differences between WTP and price across the total amount consumed.

An example of such a technology might be a childhood vaccination program in which one "shot" provides lifetime immunity (no "boosters" needed) and the entire population has been vaccinated. In this situation, there is no further ability to adjust on extensive or intensive margins. At this point, the ICER may be well below the decision threshold.

MODELS OF PHARMACEUTICAL (AND RELATED) PRICING

The distinction between "price" and "value" arises because only a very few medical care markets operate under the conditions resembling pure competition that are taught in introductory economics classes. In those highly simplified models, price has a very different meaning. At the intersection of a market demand curve and a market supply curve, it measures both the marginal costs of production (the height of the industry supply curve) and the marginal value of consumption (the height of the demand curve) at the intersection of the two.

For the most part, producers in health care markets have some form of market power, allowing them to raise prices above marginal costs of production. Numerous models of market equilibrium exist to describe how price is set under various noncompetitive conditions. The pure monopoly is the simplest of these. In this world, producers find the quantity of output that maximizes profits, the amount where added revenue ("marginal revenue") equals added costs ("marginal costs") if one additional unit of output is produced. Then monopolists set prices that "clear the market." Such prices always exceed the marginal costs of production.

One useful and intuitive measure of monopoly power was created by Lerner (1934). It states that the extent of monopoly power can be measured by the proportion of price that is due to "markup" above marginal cost. The Lerner index is $\Lambda = \dfrac{\text{Price} - \text{Marginal Cost}}{\text{Price}}$. One feature of this analysis is that for a profit-maximizing monopolist, $\Lambda = \dfrac{1}{|\eta|}$, so the smaller the demand elasticity, η, the greater the markup.

In a market in which a drug company sets a single price, the question becomes how to set the socially optimal markup—a question first answered in a model developed by economist Frank Ramsey (1927).[1] Ramsey's model seeks to find the price that balances the incentives toward lower cost (to make the drugs more affordable for consumers) with incentive for innovation. Instead of using the Lerner index, $\Lambda = \dfrac{1}{|\eta|}$, as the pricing rule, these "Ramsey-rule" methods set the optimal price as $P^* = \dfrac{k}{|\eta|}$, where $0 < k < 1$, and k is chosen through various methods to balance the competing goals of affordability and innovation.

In most developed countries, however, the pricing of biopharmaceutical products departs from Ramsey's approach due to prescription drug insurance. Health insurance reduces the demand elasticity for the insured goods and services (Phelps, 2018, Chapter 11). Moreover, health insurance decouples the price paid to the drug manufacturer from the price paid by the consumer. Third-party payers bargain with manufacturers over what price the payer will pay to the manufacturer. Separately, the payer (or its agents) will set cost sharing for beneficiaries such that the consumers' shares will be much less than prices paid to manufacturers.

With health insurance coverage, the demand elasticity will continue to influence how insured consumers respond to changes in co-payments. However, when prices are bargained between drug companies and third-party payers, the underlying market demand elasticity is no longer relevant to price-setting (Lakdawalla and Sood, 2013). What matters instead are the degrees of bargaining leverage possessed by the drug company and its payer counterpart. At the limit, when drug companies possess all the bargaining power, prices will be equal to the total expected value that consumers assign to the drug. In practice, even a drug company with total bargaining leverage will receive less than this because inefficiencies associated with moral hazard, adverse selection, and other insurance market frictions will ultimately take bites out of its revenues (Lakdawalla and Sood, 2013). Moreover, third-party payers often have leverage too, which reduces the drug companies' share of value further.

Evidently, in a price-bargaining equilibrium, drug companies will receive some share of the value of their product, where the share depends on
their bargaining leverage vis-à-vis the third-party payer and on frictions
in the health insurance marketplace. But what share of value *should* they
receive? This is a question that has not so far been satisfactorily resolved
by economists. In looking at the Ramsey markup method, where $P^* = \dfrac{k}{|\eta|}$
and $0 < k < 1$, no clear methods have emerged to determine the optimal
level of k.

In 1969, the economist William Nordhaus published what became
known as the Nordhaus model of innovation (Nordhaus, 1969a, 1969b).
He contends that innovators decide how much to invest in research by
maximizing their expected profits. An important implication is that greater
rewards for innovation will stimulate more research and more innovation,
an empirical prediction that has since been validated many times over in
the economics literature (Acemoglu and Linn, 2004; Finkelstein, 2004;
Blume-Kohout and Sood, 2013; Dubois et al., 2015).

More controversial was an important normative implication of his
model: The Nordhaus model concludes that the level of innovation is efficient when innovators receive the entirety of the value they create with
their innovation. Among other things, this would imply that the net monetary benefits of new innovations ought always to be 0, if innovation is
efficiently provided.

Subsequent research demonstrated the fragility of this result. Among
the more well-known critiques is that advanced by Glenn Loury (1979).
He argues that when innovators compete to discover new inventions, the
resulting "patent races" can result in duplication of effort and too much
entry into innovation. His solution is for innovators to receive less than
the full value of their inventions, but how much less remains unclear.

To be sure, there are some undesirable features of Loury's (1979) approach
when applied to the pharmaceutical industry. Notably, he assumes a "winner-
take-all" model in which the first firm to discover a new technology earns
all the profits from it. In the pharmaceutical industry, on the other hand, it
can be quite profitable to bring the second, third, or later drug in the class

to market, even before expiration of the first innovator's patent. Regardless, Loury points out that Nordhaus's policy implication ignores interactions among competitive firms. Unfortunately, Loury's approach leaves the literature in the dark about how much value innovators should receive.

Socially efficient prices for innovation have so far eluded economic theorists (Lakdawalla, 2018). However, all is not lost. Calls for value-based pricing recognize Nordhaus's key empirical implication that prices cannot be driven down to marginal cost without destroying incentives for innovation. Therefore, price-setting models for prescription drugs seek out methods with three properties. First, more valuable products command higher prices and vice versa. This is the point where the choice of valuation method (standard CEA or GRACE) would matter most. Second, innovators earn profits to sustain their incentives for innovation. Third, efficient pricing distributes the costs of innovation in ways that maximize access for all the patients who derive value in excess of marginal cost of production.

These criteria provide some guidance about international price comparisons. They state that countries with higher WTP for pharmaceuticals should pay higher prices. In many cases, this works out in a way such that wealthier countries pay higher prices and hence bear the greatest burden in financing innovation in the biopharmaceutical industry (Danzon et al., 2015).

We can also assess issues of "who pays" for innovation under current systems. Under current approaches to incentivizing research and development, current users of prescription drugs effectively pay for future development.[2] In a world with no insurance for purchase of these drugs, many people might view this as wholly unfair. Why should today's "sick" patients pay for tomorrow's innovation?

However, with widespread prescription drug insurance, all enrollees in the insurance collectively pay for the use of "today's" drugs, whose prices also happen to influence biopharmaceutical innovators' expectations about prices in the future. This does not clarify the socially efficient pricing level (i.e., how large of a "markup" above marginal cost is appropriate), but it at least allays concerns about the inequity of today's sickest patients also bearing the burden of tomorrow's research.

Of course, this analysis only applies with widespread or universal insurance for prescription drugs, a situation that is obviously not wholly present in the United States. Those who pay high prices for today's drugs but have no prescription drug insurance would certainly not agree that the current system is fair and equitable. The solution to this conundrum does not so much lie in the domain of pricing for prescription drugs as in the public policy area of access to prescription drug insurance.

With that statement "off our chests," we turn naturally to the question of how best to measure value when seeking to align "prices" of medical interventions to value created by their use. This matters either in market-based environments (e.g., the United States), where "price" is explicitly negotiated between insurance plans and health care providers, or in centralized national systems such as the British National Health Service, where formal CEA methods provide a backdrop for price negotiations. "We note here that the 2022 Inflation Reduction Act (IRA) requires that the Centers for Medicare and Medicaid Services (CMS) begin negotiations for prescription drugs, and requires them to include "value" as part of their pricing determinations. At the same time the IRA and preceding Affordable Care Act (ACA) preclude CMS from using standard CEA methods, since they discriminate against disabled people. We believe that GRACE allows CMS to comply both with the requirement to measure value of prescription drugs and at the same time not discriminate against disabled people. This could become an important issue in US healthcare policy.

VALUE WHEN CHANGING FROM STANDARD CEA TO GRACE

As noted in the Preface, GRACE changes the way value is measured in five distinct ways: (1) Value for treatments of low-severity diseases falls; (2) value for treatments of high-severity diseases rises at a faster-than-linear rate; (3) value for treating people with disability rises with the degree of disability, a stark reversal of standard CEA methods; (4) uncertainty in treatment outcomes affects value; and (5) the willingness to trade LE and HRQoL varies with baseline health status, unlike standard CEA methods in which this trade-off rate is the same for all levels of baseline HRQoL and LE.

As we have previously noted in Chapters 2–6, if analysts are willing to assume a specific utility function for $W(H)$, then the key GRACE parameters can be computed directly. Appendix 6.1 shows the details of this approach. In what follows, we assume that analysts prefer to avoid assuming a specific utility function, and we use the Taylor series approximations discussed in previous chapters. Encompassing all these changes in summary measures of value is a complex enterprise, too much to explore in complete detail. The remainder of this chapter explores what we believe are the key features of GRACE as it might apply to a health insurer's or health plan's measure of the value that it creates and (where applicable) how this might affect prices negotiated between health insurers and providers. This type of negotiation is, of course, almost universally applicable in the domains of prescription drugs and medical devices, where both health insurers (as in the United States) and universal health plans (as in the United Kingdom) directly purchase biopharmaceutical products from external producers. We therefore attempt to provide a guide for thinking about consequences for insurers in market-based environments and health plan providers where comprehensive (and perhaps universal) care is provided. In order to cut down on complexity, we set aside issues of disability in what follows, setting $D = 1$.

First-Order Effects

INTRODUCTION

To begin, we need some simplifying assumptions. Our first assumptions are that the demographic and health characteristics of the enrolled health insurance population are stable over time. The next assumption is that the available treatment technology remains unchanged. Although technological change is evident in health care, it is still useful to calculate spending for a given level of technology. In this framework, we can characterize the mix of patients who receive treatments as a function of the health technology assessment (HTA) decision rules used by the health system. For this discussion, we assume that HTA is based on standard CEA and that payments to providers (if a third-party insurer) vary with the value assessments of this HTA process. In the first-order sequence of shifting to a GRACE-based valuation system, we envision that clinicians will continue to treat patients the same way, even though reimbursements might vary according to disease severity (ℓ^*) and other GRACE-related considerations.

With a stable population mix, a stable set of available technologies, and a stable set of treatment recommendations (protocol-based or merely standard patterns of treatment), then one can define a percentage (share) of all treatments accounted for by any treatment, j, as s_j.[3]

Next, for each treatment, j, associated with it will be an untreated illness severity ℓ_j^* and an average HRQoL improvement, μ_{Bj}. The combination of these two measures leads immediately to an average R value, $\overline{R_j}$, associated with each treatment $j = 1 \ldots J$. The computation for this value directly follows the methods defined in Chapter 2, using the integrated Taylor series expansion shown in Eq. (11.1), a repetition here (for convenience) of Eq. (2.11b):[4]

$$\overline{R}_j \approx \int_a^b R(\ell^*)d\ell^* = \ell^* + \frac{1}{2!}r^*\ell^{*2} + \frac{1}{3!}r_H^*\pi_H^*\ell^{*3} + \frac{1}{4!}r_H^*\pi_H^*\tau_H^*\ell^{*4} + \ldots \quad (11.1)$$

where a and b respectively are the pre- and post-treatment values of ℓ^* involved for treatment j.

To use Table 2.2 for incremental (nonmarginal) cures, one should first choose the appropriate level of r_H^* to get onto the proper row. Estimates of these should be available from researchers, and they do not need to be estimated for each HTA. Then, for any particular medical intervention j, one must know the severity level for untreated disease, ℓ^*, and the extent of health improvement provided, μ_{Bj}. To obtain the average R value for intervention j, find the $\overline{R}_j$ value for the untreated illness, and then the value (along the same row) for the treated illness, which is defined as $\ell_j^* - \mu_{Bj}$. Their difference provides the total value of treatment using the R multiplier, and the average can be found by dividing the total R-weighted quality-adjusted life year (QALY) gain by the actual QALY gain created by the intervention, μ_{Bj}.

To provide a precise example, assume that $r_H^* = 0.7$, and that the untreated illness has a value of $\ell_j^* = 0.7$. If intervention j improves health by 0.5 on a scale from 0 to 1.0, (i.e., $\mu_{Bj} = 0.5$), then the treated value is

Table 11.1 INTEGRAL VALUES FOR VARIOUS DEGREES OF ILLNESS SEVERITY AND
RELATIVE RISK AVERSION[a]

| | Illness Severity | | | | | | | | |
r^*	0.1	0.2	0.3	0.4	0.5	0.6	0.7	0.8	0.9
0	0.1	0.2	0.3	0.4	0.5	0.6	0.7	0.8	0.9
0.1	0.10	0.20	0.31	0.41	0.51	0.62	0.73	0.84	0.97
0.2	0.10	0.20	0.31	0.42	0.53	0.65	0.77	0.91	1.05
0.3	0.10	0.21	0.32	0.43	0.55	0.68	0.81	0.97	1.14
0.4	0.10	0.21	0.32	0.44	0.57	0.71	0.86	1.03	1.25
0.5	0.10	0.21	0.33	0.45	0.59	0.74	0.90	1.11	1.36
0.6	0.10	0.21	0.34	0.46	0.61	0.77	0.96	1.19	1.50
0.7	0.10	0.22	0.34	0.47	0.63	0.80	1.01	1.28	1.66
0.8	0.10	0.22	0.33	0.49	0.65	0.84	1.06	1.38	1.84
0.9	0.11	0.22	0.35	0.50	0.67	0.88	1.13	1.49	2.04
1	0.11	0.23	0.36	0.51	0.69	0.92	1.20	1.61	2.28

[a]Estimates of average $\overline{R}_j$ for various levels of ℓ^*, μ_B, and r_H^*. Along any row (fixed r_H^*), the difference between any two values of ℓ^* indicates the average health gain, μ_B. This table uses Taylor series methods (see Eq. 11.1) to obtain values. For results using the numerical integration approach, see Table 2.2.

$\ell_j^* = 0.2$. Table 11.1 tells us that the value of this improvement is (1.01 – 0.22) = 0.79 units of gain in HRQoL. This value is created by an intervention that created an improvement of 0.5 QALYs. Therefore, the average value per unit of HRQoL gain is 0.79/0.5 = 1.58. For this intervention, the value created is 1.58 units of HRQoL gain times the WTP value of K_{GRACE}, ignoring any changes in the random outcomes of T and C (i.e., that $\varepsilon = 1$). Later, we discuss how to incorporate values of ε if they are available, or the proper process if the analysis assumes that $\varepsilon = 1$.

MEASURING AGGREGATE VALUE CHANGES

As we now demonstrate, the concepts in Table 11.1, combined with measures of the average HRQoL improvement and average untreated illness severity, will usefully illuminate how shifting to a GRACE-based system will affect overall measures of value in any health plan.

Define H_{1j} as the treated health level in period 1 associated with treatment j. Similarly, define P_j as the fraction of period 1 of which patients are expected to live, post-treatment, and define μ_{P_j} as the change in that fraction post-treatment. When using standard CEA, where H_1, the treated health level in period 1, is the marginal rate of substitution between LE and HRQoL, the total value provided across all $j = 1 \ldots J$ treatments provided by the health plan in period 1 (each with a share s_j) is

$$TV_{\mathrm{CEA}} = KJ\sum_{j=1}^{J} s_j (H_{1j}\mu_{Pj} + P_j\mu_{Bj}) \tag{11.2a}$$

Similarly, where ρ_j is discussed in Chapter 4, the total value under GRACE is given by

$$TV_{\mathrm{GRACE}} = KJ\sum_{j=1}^{J} s_j (\rho_j\mu_{Pj} + P_j\omega_H \overline{R}_j\mu_{Bj}\varepsilon_j) \tag{11.2b}$$

As Chapter 4 demonstrates, GRACE treats extensions in LE similarly to the way they are treated in standard CEA. Therefore, as a first-order approximation, we believe that in most cases, the value of changes in LE under GRACE will not change markedly from the valuation created with standard CEA.

Because of these various factors, for the immediate first-order approximation, we focus on the difference in valuation created for improvements in HRQoL. Without loss of generality, we define VE_0 as the valuation effect per period of survival; therefore, we normalize $P_j = 1$, which causes the P_j terms to drop out. Hence, the first-order valuation effect, VE_0, is

$$VE_0 = KJ\sum_{j=1}^{J} s_j\omega_H \overline{R}_j\varepsilon_j\mu_{Bj} - KJ\sum_{j=1}^{J} s_j\mu_{Bj} \tag{11.3}$$

Now define a combined valuation for each technology, $\Phi_j \equiv \omega_H \overline{R}_j\varepsilon_j$, a valuation that can ultimately be characterized for each technology. Clearly,

Φ_j is a combination of known (or knowable) features for each technology $j = 1, \ldots J$, the values of μ_{Bj} and ε_j, and the (currently unknown) risk preference parameters, ω_H, r_H^*, π_H^*, and higher order risk parameters as needed to estimate $\overline{R}_j$. Calculating ε_j also requires knowing relevant populations' risk-preference parameters for use according to Eq. (3.1).

Once the necessary risk-preference parameters are known, one can readily calculate each $\overline{R}_j$ using the methods described in Chapter 2. In addition to the risk-preference parameters, this requires knowing, for each technology $j = 1, \ldots J$, average ℓ_j^* values and mean HRQoL gains, μ_{Bj}.

With these simplifying assumptions, the first-order value effect, VE_0, becomes

$$VE_0 = KJ\sum_{j=1}^{J}s\mu_{Bj}(\Phi_j - 1) \tag{11.4}$$

Three key elements determine VE_0: the value measures, Φ_j; the shares of treatments provided by the health care agency, s; and the average treatment benefit, μ_{Bj}. The initial distribution of treatments (s_j) can be readily determined by any insurer or health care provider from their medical records and/or insurance claims systems. Next, μ_{Bj} represents the average HRQoL gains produced by treatments.

Finally, $(\Phi_j - 1)$ represents the differential value placed on each treatment by GRACE, compared with standard CEA. It is important to note that some combinations of the relevant parameters lead to situations in which $\overline{\Phi} < 1$. Simulations that follow shortly demonstrate this phenomenon. In these cases, valuation by K_{GRACE} is lower than when using standard CEA methods.

Recall that $\Phi_j \equiv \varepsilon_j\omega_H\overline{R}_j$. We think it likely that initial efforts to use GRACE will assess the value of existing medical interventions retrospectively. In doing so, we assume that they will set $\varepsilon = 1$, then that leaves the key value measures, $\omega_H\overline{R}_j$. Since $\overline{R}_j$ depends on the risk-preference parameters, r_H^* and higher order terms, this focuses our attention on how ω_H and r_H^* interact. Once we know these two terms, we can determine all of the risk-preference terms needed to calculate $\overline{R}_j$, and hence the key products $\omega_H \overline{R}_j$ for each technology, $j = 1, \ldots J$, offered by the health plan.

This set of calculations cannot be done immediately. However, we know from Chapter 2 that $\overline{R}_j$ will not diverge notably from a value of 1 for many treatments—those where the untreated illness severity is low and, most particularly, where both the untreated illness, ℓ^*, and the treatment effect, μ_{Bj}, are small. However, we also know that $\overline{R}_j$ substantially exceeds 1.0 for many important medical interventions.

As health plans seek to understand the consequences of shifting from standard CEA (or less formal methods of valuation) to GRACE, their first order of business to estimate VE_0 should focus on estimating Φ_j for the most important treatments offered by a health plan (taking into account the share of the total, s_j, the average HRQoL gain from treatment, and some assessment of the untreated illness severity so that Φ_j can be estimated).

We also note that the set of $(\Phi_j - 1)$ values can plausibly be "done once" and may not have to be done by each health plan. The application of technologies to illnesses, although not uniform throughout their own nation, can plausibly be estimated at least initially by first using national averages of ℓ^*_j and μ_{Bj} for each technology, thus obtaining national averages for each $\overline{R}_j$.

Individual health plans may well find that their own pertinent values will diverge from national averages for several reasons. The most likely of these involves different decision-making processes on the extensive and intensive margins about the appropriate population for which each treatment $j = 1, \ldots J$ is appropriate (Phelps, 1997). Widely documented regional variations in the use of various medical technologies suggest that these regional differences could be important (Phelps, 2000) and could significantly alter the allocation of resources within a health plan (represented by the treatment shares, s_j); the average untreated illness severity, ℓ^*_j; and the average HRQoL benefit, μ_{Bj}.

Whether done nationally, regionally, or in separate health plans, for many technologies, good information about treatment benefits, including mean benefits, can be ascertained from extant CEA studies in the

Tufts University database. Given that most of these studies do not report variances or higher order risk terms, initial computation to measure VE_0 may well need to assume that $\varepsilon_j = 1$ for most technologies.

The Dance Involving ω_H and r_H^*

BACKGROUND

As Chapter 2 suggests, ω_H and r_H^* move in a rhythmic dance. In the simplest (yet reasonably plausible) case, we have constant relative risk aversion (CRRA) so that $\omega_H + r_H^* = 1$. When one goes down, the other goes up. Looking at Eq. (11.5), and remembering that $\Phi_j \equiv \varepsilon_j \omega_H \overline{R}_j$, one can see that this plays itself out in the product of $\omega_H \times \overline{R}_j$, which will largely determine whether net treatment valuations are positive or negative, and the magnitude of each $\overline{R}_j$ will depend on the mix of patients covered by any given health plan and the burden of illness they bring with them. To explore these issues, we next develop a series of simulations showing how various combinations of ω_H and r_H^* can affect the net valuations by health plans of their portfolio of medical interventions upon their adoption of GRACE.

SIMULATIONS

Low-Severity Illnesses

We do not explore values of $\Phi_j = \varepsilon_j \omega_H \overline{R}_j$ with low initial illness severity for a very simple reason: The value of R does not diverge far from 1.0 for low-severity illnesses. Looking at Table 11.1, one can see that for illness severity at $\ell^* = 0.1$, the $\overline{R}_j$ values are essentially identical when $r_H^* = 0$, the appropriate value when using standard CEA, when $r_H^* = 1$, and for all intervening values of r_H^*. GRACE differs only by 10 percent from standard CEA valuation in this range. The same observation holds for combinations of r_H^* and ℓ^* where both are relatively small. For all practical purposes, only in the lower right half (the lower diagonal) of Table 11.1 do the GRACE integral values substantially exceed the comparable standard CEA values (which appear in the top row of Table 11.1, where $r_H^* = 0$).

Sensitivity Analysis

To begin this exercise, we choose a value of $\omega_H = 0.5$ and hold it fixed. For these different "cases," we will also set $\omega_C = 0.5$ so that $K = \dfrac{C}{\omega_C} = 2C$. Thus, "2" becomes the standard CEA multiplier of C for comparison purposes.

In all of these examples, the values shown are the *marginal* values from Table 2.1, not the average values from Table 2.2 or Table 11.1. For actual analyses of value changes, it will be necessary to measure the incremental gain in health for each intervention j and derive the appropriate $\overline{R}_j$ values from Table 11.1 (using the Taylor series values) or Table 2.2 (using the numerical integration values). The examples that follow (using marginal values) are intended to demonstrate the consequences of using different patterns of ω_H and r_H^*.

Remember that all of these examples are hypothetical because no measure yet exists of r_H^* or ω_H, or how they might vary as H changes. This analysis applies the use of hyperbolic absolute risk aversion (HARA) utility functions as discussed in Chapter 8.

Case 1: CRRA utility with $\omega_H + r^* = 1$

As a baseline, we assume the easiest situation to analyze—where $W(H)$ is CRRA so that $\omega_H + r_H^* = 1$. This is a good starting point, from which we can depart in several directions to see how the results change as the key parameters, ω_H and r_H^*, change.

Table 11.2a and subsequent similar tables show in **bold font** those situations in which the K_{GRACE} multiplier exceeds 2.0, so the GRACE valuation exceeds $2C$ the relevant comparison for our simulations. With this "baseline" set of parameters, only for illness severity of approximately $\ell^* = 0.75$ and higher (interpolating between values in the second row of Table 11.2a) is the marginal R value higher in GRACE than in standard CEA, and for low-severity illnesses ($\ell^* = 0.1$), the standard

Table 11.2a M<small>ULTIPLIERS OF</small> C <small>TO</small> O<small>BTAIN</small> P<small>ROPER</small> M<small>ARGINAL</small>
K_{GRACE} V<small>ALUES</small>[a]

C<small>ASE</small> 1: $r_H^* = 0.5$, $\omega_H = 0.5$

Illness Severity

0.1	0.2	0.3	0.4	0.5	0.6	0.7	0.8	0.9
1.05	1.12	1.20	1.29	1.41	1.58	1.83	**2.24**	**3.16**

[a]CEA comparison multipliers equal 2.0.

CEA value is almost cut in half, a direct result of having assumed that $\omega_H = 0.5$ compared with the standard CEA assumption that $\omega_H = 1.0$.

Next, we explore two non-CRRA possible situations, one in which $r_H^* + \omega_H = 1.3$ and another in which $r_H^* + \omega_H = 0.7$. Both are possible, the first with decreasing relative risk aversion (DRRA) and the latter having increasing relative risk aversion (IRRA), rather than the previous assumption that utility was CRRA. These two examples both have the same "shift" away from the CRRA case in which $r_H^* + \omega_H = 1$, to demonstrate symmetrically how the overall effect of GRACE changes as these key risk parameters change.

Case 2: $r_H^* + \omega_H = 1.3$

Since (by assumption for the example $\omega_H = 0.5$), this means that $r_H^* = 0.8$. Reading off of Table 2.1 for $r_H^* = 0.8$, the severity levels are in row 1 and the marginal severity multipliers (R) are in row 2.

The second row of Table 11.2b (the values of R) gives the proper multiplier for consumption, C, since we have assumed that $\omega_H = \omega_C = 0.5$. In this specific case, $K_{\text{GRACE}} = \left[\dfrac{\omega_H}{\omega_C} \right] RC = RC$. With this specific assumption about the levels of r_H^* and ω_H, the "multiplier" for C is greater than 2.0 for illness severity levels from just a bit under $\ell^* = 0.6$ to higher severity levels (as highlighted in bold). The multiplier exceeds 6.0 for the highest-severity illnesses ($\ell^* = 0.9$), more than triple the value in standard CEA for these parameter assumptions. However, for $\ell^* < 0.6$, multipliers are less

Table 11.2b MULTIPLIERS OF *C* TO OBTAIN PROPER MARGINAL
K_{GRACE} VALUES[a]

CASE 2: $r_H^* = 0.8$, $\omega_H = 0.5$.

Illness Severity (ℓ^*)								
0.1	0.2	0.3	0.4	0.5	0.6	0.7	0.8	0.9
1.09	1.2	1.33	1.5	1.74	**2.08**	**2.62**	**3.62**	**6.35**

[a]CEA comparison multipliers equal 2.0.

than 2.0, in which case the GRACE valuation is lower than the standard CEA valuation (again, given the parameter assumptions). As in the CRRA situation, total system valuation will rise or fall depending on the mix of illness severity in the covered population. With the assumptions in Table 11.2b, an increase in valuation when using GRACE occurs more readily than in the CRRA situation, but the basic answer will still apply: It depends on the patient illness mix and (when calculating actual treatment gains) the magnitudes of each μ_{Bj} in a health plan's portfolio of treatments.

Case 3: $r_H^* + \omega_H = 0.7$

Now consider the opposite situation in which utility is IRRA, and $r_H^* + \omega_H = 0.7$. This is symmetric to Case 1 except that utility is IRRA, but of the same degree of shift away from CRRA as was Case 2. Here, in Case 3, since $\omega_H = 0.5$, and $r_H^* + \omega_H = 0.7$, then $r^* = 0.2$. Now we can read off the *R* multipliers from the proper row of Table 2.1.

Table 11.2c MULTIPLIERS OF *C* TO OBTAIN PROPER MARGINAL
K_{GRACE} VALUES[a]

CASE 3: $r_H^* = 0.2$, $\omega_H = 0.5$.

Illness Severity								
0.1	0.2	0.3	0.4	0.5	0.6	0.7	0.8	0.9
1.02	1.05	1.07	1.11	1.15	1.2	1.27	1.38	1.57

[a]CEA comparison multipliers equal 2.0.

In this example, *every* marginal valuation is lower using GRACE methods than the standard CEA model for this set of parameters—that is, $K = 2C$. With these assumed risk-preference parameters, total valuations will assuredly fall if that health system switches from standard CEA to GRACE valuation methods.

Case 4: $r_H^* + \omega_H = 1.3$ (again)[5]

A third alternative to CRRA might arise, where $r_H^* + \omega_H > 1$ but the "excess" in the sum of the two preference parameters alters ω_H, not r_H^*. To continue with the example, again suppose (as in Case 2) that $r_H^* + \omega_H = 1.3$ but now with $r_H^* = 0.5$ and $\omega_H = 0.8$. Then the basic multiplier is $\dfrac{\omega_H}{\omega_C} = \dfrac{0.8}{0.5} = 1.6$. Now, with $r_H^* = 0.5$, the results are shown in Table 11.2d. This differs from Case 1 in a simple way: All values in row 2 of Table 11.2d are multiplied by a factor of 1.6 because we are now assuming that $\dfrac{\omega_H}{\omega_C} = 1.6$, not 1.0.

In Case 4, all illness levels above severity of about $\ell^* = 0.35$ (again, interpolating between values in row 2 of Table 11.2d) have K_{GRACE} values that exceed the CEA value of $K = 2C$. Compared with Case 2, the value gradient is flatter, even though in both cases $r_H^* + \omega_H = 1.3$. In Case 2, when $\ell^* = 0.9$, the multiplier is $R = 7.91$. In Case 4, $R = 5.06$. But at the low end of severity, Case 4 has higher valuations than does Case 2. In Table 11.2d (Case 4), system total values would very likely rise unless the patient mix was tilted strongly toward low-severity illnesses.

Table 11.2d Multipliers of C to Obtain Proper Marginal K_{GRACE} Values[a]

Case 4: $r_H^* = 0.5,\ \omega_H = 0.8$.

Illness Severity								
0.1	0.2	0.3	0.4	0.5	0.6	0.7	0.8	0.9
1.68	1.79	1.92	2.06	2.26	2.53	2.93	3.58	5.06

[a]CEA comparison multipliers equal 2.0.

The differences shown in Tables 11.2a–11.2d (using marginal R values) point out the high level of importance of understanding whether risk aversion is IRRA, CRRA, or DRRA and the magnitude of the relevant parameters. These situations lead to *very* different valuations for medical interventions, both in the level of the valuations and in the steepness of the value gradient. Comparable differences will arise when calculating average severity-adjustment values, the $\overline{R}_j$, that are necessary to compute each $(\Phi_j - 1)$.

Analyzing Discrete (Versus Marginal) Changes in Value

We earlier noted that the previous simulations use "marginal" R values, whereas the complete analysis of the effect of shifting from standard CEA to GRACE must take into account average values of QALY gains, expressed as $\overline{R}_j$ for each intervention j. Although the various permutations of possibilities would overwhelm our ability to demonstrate all of these effects, in this section we provide several examples of how to conduct this final step.

A simple "bottom line" emerges from these considerations: Shifting from marginal values, R, to average values, $\overline{R}_j$, "flattens out" the distinction between standard CEA and GRACE to some extent. The reason is simple: The two methods differ by only small amounts for low-severity illnesses, so calculating the value of a "complete cure" brings into the analysis a range of severity levels (in the integral from ℓ^* to t^* —that is, from untreated illness to treated illness), where GRACE and standard CEA values have little difference.

We use two examples of different "technologies" to demonstrate this phenomenon. The first example measures the value of an intervention that improves the HRQoL for a very sick person from $\ell^* = 0.9$ to 0.7, an important gain in HRQoL but nevertheless not a complete cure. The second intervention begins at the same low HRQoL, $\ell^* = 0.9$, but provides a complete cure, bringing health to a normal level of H_0. We do this for the same combinations of parameters used in Cases 1–4 in the preceding section. We compare the valuations of each of these interventions using both GRACE and standard CEA for these four sets of GRACE-related parameters. In all of these cases, we use $\omega_C = 0.5$ so $K = 2C$ for each full QALY gained.

Case 1: CRRA with r_H^* and ω_H both equal to 0.5

In these examples, we use Table 11.1, which provides $\overline{R}$ values for various combinations of r_H^* and ℓ^*. This exercise will also remind readers about how to use Table 11.1 (or the numerical integration equivalent, Table 2.2).

The "partial cure" intervention improves health from $\ell^* = 0.9$ to 0.7, a moderate improvement from a very low untreated HRQoL. Reading from Table 11.1 along the row where $r_H^* = 0.5$, the relevant entries are 1.36 (for $\ell^* = 0.9$) and 0.9 (for $\ell^* = 0.7$), so the "value score" is $1.36 - 0.9 = 0.46$ for a 0.2 QALY gain, or an average gain of 2.3 per QALY. The 0.46 value—the product of $\overline{R}_j$ and μ_{Bj} in Eq. (11.3)—is the one that "counts." With $\omega_H = 0.5$ and $\omega_C = 0.5$, $K_{\text{GRACE}} = 1 \times C$, and the total value gained is $0.46 \times C$. With standard CEA, the value gained would be 0.2 QALYs times $2C$ per QALY, or $0.40 \times C$. GRACE shows a higher valuation than standard CEA, but not by much.

Now consider the "full cure" technology in the same situation. Again, the WTP in GRACE (with the assumed utility parameters) is C per QALY. From Table 11.1, a full cure from $\ell^* = 0.9$ creates a total value of 1.36 QALYs, and hence a WTP of $1.36 \times C$. However, standard CEA, which (as we have argued) overvalues low-severity health gains, would value this total cure at 0.9 QALYs $\times$ $2C$ per QALY, for a total value of $1.80 \times C$.

Case 2: DRRA with $r_H^* = 0.8$, $\omega_H = 0.5$

This calculation is the same as in Case 1, except that we read off the row of Table 11.1 at $r_H^* = 0.8$, not 0.5. The GRACE values for the "partial cure" are 1.84 and 1.06, for a gain of 0.78 QALYs. Valued at C per QALY (as in Case 1), the net gain is $0.78 \times C$. The standard CEA comparator is the same as in Case 1, with a value of $0.40 \times C$. In this case, the GRACE valuation is almost twice that of the standard CEA valuation. The difference from Case

1 arises because of the greater value of r_H^*, which leads to higher values of R and $\bar{R}$.

The "complete cure" with $r_H^* = 0.8$ is 1.84 QALYs gained at a value of C per QALY, for a total of $1.84 \times C$. Here, with a gain of 0.9 QALYs, the standard CEA valuation is 0.9 QALYs $\times 2C = 1.8C$. The two methods are nearly equivalent in this situation.

Case 3: $r_H^* = 0.2$, $\omega_H = 0.5$.

This case is not very interesting. We already know from Table 11.2c that the marginal values are lower for GRACE than for standard CEA at all levels of r_H^* and ℓ^*, so the consequent $\bar{R}$ values are necessarily lower. We leave the exact calculation as an exercise for the reader.

Case 4: $r_H^* = 0.5$, $\omega_H = 0.8$.

This case is a mix of Cases 1 and 2. For the partial cure, we return to the QALY gain of 0.46 QALYs, only with ω_H now equal to 0.8, the K_{GRACE} basic multiplier is $\dfrac{\omega_H}{\omega_C} = \dfrac{0.8}{0.5} = 1.6C$, so the total value gain is 0.46 QALYs valued at $1.6C$, for a total of $0.74 \times C$. Again, as a reminder, the standard CEA valuation in this situation is $0.40 \times C$.

Finally, we turn to the "total cure" valuation with this set of utility parameters. With GRACE, the total QALY gain is 1.36 QALYs, the valuation is $1.6C$ per QALY, for a total value gain of $2.176 \times C$. Again, as a reminder, the standard CEA reference value for the "full cure" is $1.8 \times C$.

Wrap-Up

The previous comparisons show the same relationships to one another as the original comparisons of Case 1 through Case 4 using marginal values. We can now see, however, that sharp differences between standard CEA and GRACE persist for "partial cure" technologies, but less distinct differences occur for "total cures." And of course, the magnitude of these differences depends importantly on the parameter values as they differ for Cases 1–4.

These results should not be surprising. Taking GRACE values as the "gold standard," we can see readily that standard CEA overvalues treatment at low levels of severity and undervalues it at high levels of severity. The overvaluation at low levels of severity pulls together the valuations for "total cure" technologies using standard CEA and GRACE, whereas the distinct valuation differences persist for the "partial cure" technologies that have effects only at higher severity values.

Longer Run Considerations

Once plans have in hand the GRACE valuations of their therapies, we expect the "product mix," the s_j values, to change, even among the existing set of technologies. Some with apparent high value in standard CEA will diminish in value, and their use will be withdrawn or shifted to lower and more efficient levels of use (along the extensive or intensive margins). Some will gain in value, and their use should be expanded, and some technologies not currently in use will become sufficiently attractive using GRACE methods to include them in the scope of benefits. Rational allocation of health care resources should lead to adjustments among alternative therapies and perhaps even withdrawal of some procedures that appear to have substantially less value under GRACE evaluation than when using standard CEA methods.

Operationally, we believe that the best process for shifting to GRACE will begin by assessing procedures that have high levels of expenditure, high levels of illness severity, and high variability in treatment outcomes. These are the types of procedures that are likely to have their apparent value change most under a shift from standard CEA methods to GRACE.

Prioritizing procedures to be "first in line" for re-evaluation may require a combination of intuition and data. What is required, in some sense, is an a priori estimate of average values of each ($\Phi_j - 1$). Several models have been developed to guide prioritization for technology assessment that can guide these efforts. One approach (Phelps and Parente, 1990; Phelps and Mooney, 1992) assesses the combination of medical spending on an intervention and geographic variability in its use, based on concepts involving the economics of information.[6] This approach was broadly accepted and woven into a method for priority setting for HTA from the Institute of Medicine[7] (Donaldson and Sox, 1992). The same concepts may be useful in prioritizing new GRACE assessments of value to compare with past CEA assessments. These assessments can readily include changes in LE to refine the analyses if such changes have been omitted from "first-round" assessments.

Longest Run Considerations

In the economists' proverbial "long run," all aspects of production processes are fungible and flexible. In the case of health plans treating patients, the long run will importantly include introduction of new technologies and removal of old ones.[8]

We hope (and believe) that widespread use of GRACE methodologies will shift the mix of innovation research to provide greater emphasis to treatment of the most severe illnesses. No matter what the extent to which this occurs, new technologies will emerge and will require valuation of their results by some process or another. As GRACE gains wider footing, increasingly more often, the initial evaluation will include GRACE methods.

SUMMARY

Until the properties of the utility function $W(H)$ are known (in terms of key parameters ω_H, r_H^*, and higher order risk preference parameters), it is not possible to assess how overall measures of value within any health plan might change. To the extent that prices (negotiated or otherwise) follow these value measures at least in a general parallel fashion, the same can be said about effects on budgets: We just do not know yet. In particular, the comparisons in Tables 11 .2a–11.2d show how markedly valuations depend on these risk-preference parameters. Perhaps the most centrally important information is whether risk aversion is constant (CRRA), increasing in health (IRRA), or decreasing in health (DRRA).

This is an odd outcome for economists to consider, because very seldom (if ever) in other situations does the elasticity of an elasticity matter. Recall here that ω_H is the elasticity of *utility* with respect to H, and r_H^* is the elasticity of *marginal utility* with respect to H. Therefore, to fully understand how GRACE might play out, we need to know these elasticities of elasticities.

Whatever emerges when these parameters are well measured, one thing is certain: Shifting to GRACE aligns systems with people's preferences, so if valuations—and with them, budgets—go up or down, if this is done properly, welfare improves. Unless there is no risk aversion in HRQoL (which we would find very surprising indeed, given the available evidence), we can state with confidence that current valuation methods (standard CEA) do not correspond with consumers' true preferences. If that divergence is significant, continued use of CEA in its standard format reduces consumers' well-being. Following standard CEA values as guidelines for covering medical interventions or other insurance-related choices will lead to misallocation of resources.

We know also that the long-run consequence of using standard CEA to measure value distorts innovation away from consumers' true preferences. Current methods reward a given improvement in HRQoL the same, no matter whether delivered to a person with a trivially mild illness or a devastating major illness.

Current CEA methods also discriminate against disabled people, specifying that improving their HRQoL and LE are both worth less than for an otherwise-similar person without that disability. GRACE corrects that error, showing that the value of improving HRQoL for disabled people rises, not falls, with disability, and under a number of plausible conditions, the same can be said for improving LE. Again, continued use of standard CEA methods conflicts with preferences of people with declining marginal utility of HRQoL.

Welfare and Equity
Implications of GRACE

That which is not good for the swarm,
neither is it good for the bee.

—MARCUS AURELIUS (Meditations, Book VI, 54)

INTRODUCTION

Through numerous presentations of the generalized risk-adjusted cost-
effectiveness (GRACE) model, we have repeatedly been asked about the
implications of GRACE regarding issues of welfare, equity, and fairness.
This presents a challenging question because GRACE, just as previous
formalizations of cost-effectiveness analysis (CEA; Garber and Phelps,
1997), is structured around the utility-maximizing behavior of a single
"representative individual." Creating further complexity, the economic literature on welfare has struggled with the conflict between "individualism"
and the need to evaluate the welfare of society as a whole. Nonetheless,
GRACE can serve as a useful tool for analyzing the equity implications of
health interventions, and it represents an important advance over traditional cost-effectiveness in this respect.

As a starting point for discussion, we briefly review the underlying
approach to the measurement of societal welfare in economic theory.

Valuing Health. Charles E. Phelps and Darius N. Lakdawalla, Oxford University Press. © Oxford University Press 2024.
DOI: 10.1093/oso/9780197686287.003.0012

Axiomatically, economic analysis requires that we avoid "interpersonal comparisons of utility." In plainer language, this means that economists are unwilling to assert that increasing Person A's utility is more important to society than increasing Person B's utility. However, new medical technologies or health policies inevitably accrue benefits to some consumers and costs to others. There seems a pressing need to weigh these consequences and determine whose costs or benefits matter more. How can we reconcile this need against the prohibition on comparing utility across people? Welfare economics threads the needle by distinguishing between judgments about efficiency and judgments about equity.

Efficiency, or sometimes "Pareto efficiency," means that we focus only on policies or outcomes that exclude waste. For example, spending money on technologies that produce no benefit, without any controversy, is a bad idea because redirecting that money harms nobody and can likely help someone else. Economists agree that ineffective policies harm social welfare. No value judgments need to be made about how to prioritize one person's utility over that of another. A weaker criterion, Kaldor–Hicks efficiency, merely requires that the aggregate net benefits of a project to those who receive its benefits exceed the aggregate net losses of those who do not partake in the benefits.[1] This essentially forms the intellectual basis for cost–benefit analysis and CEA.

Efficiency provides a good starting point for welfare analysis, but it leaves many important questions unresolved. For example, providing a highly cost-effective technology only to the richest members of society may be just as efficient as providing it only to the poorest, even though most ordinary humans would view these two projects quite differently. Economists would describe the choice between these two policies as driven by an ethical judgment, not economic analysis. Although economic analysis does not provide mathematical tools for making this ethical decision, it does provide us with a way of making the ethical judgments transparent.

To see this specifically, we turn to the foundational work of economist John Harsanyi (1955), whose paper laid the groundwork for welfare analysis under uncertainty.[2] He showed that all efficient allocations of goods can be described as maximizing a "social welfare function," which consists of a weighted average of expected utilities. In this model, the weights on the expected utilities embed the ethical judgments about the importance placed on each person. Harsanyi's framework clearly identifies the set of efficient policies and technologies, and it also clarifies the value judgments being made.

Readers familiar with welfare economics might be surprised that we turn to Harsanyi instead of his arguably more famous peer, John Rawls. Rawls' famous work, *A Theory of Justice* (1971), argues that "just" outcomes can be reached only if agents make decisions behind a "veil of ignorance" that blinds them to their social position, status, or other personal characteristics (Adler, 2002, pp. 1274–1275). Our difficulty with Rawls is his adoption of a radical and, in our context, unwieldy approach to ex ante decision-making under uncertainty. In a Rawlsian world, decisions are made as if consumers know nothing about their probabilities of being in one state or another, a viewpoint that precludes allocating resources to uses that are likely to produce the most value.

The most specific instance of this is that our model allows our representative consumer to know both the probability of survival into the future, p, and (if surviving) the probability that any specific disease might occur, ϕ. Therefore, the Rawlsian approach is fundamentally incompatible with forward-looking consumer behavior under uncertainty. Specifically, our forward-looking model describes the total value of a medical intervention in terms of willingness to pay (WTP) in period 0 for access to a medical treatment in period 1, which requires knowledge of both the probability of survival, p_n, and the probability of the relevant disease occurring, ϕ.

To further describe Harsanyi's (1955) model of social welfare, suppose that we have a society consisting of N individuals wherein all individuals (i) derive utility from their consumption of goods and of health. For analytical simplicity, we suppose that utility functions are the same for all members of society, although levels of consumption and health might not be. Therefore, define individual i's utility as $U(C_i)W(H_i)$, as before, a "separable" utility function. Now define some set of welfare weights, θ_i, where $\sum_{i=1}^{N}\theta_i = 1$. Generally speaking, θ_i is the relative importance placed upon individual i in our ethical approach to welfare. These weights cannot be determined by economic analysis. They involve ethical, philosophical, or political choices.

Harsanyi (1955) shows that for some chosen set of welfare weights, maximizing the weighted sum of expected utilities produces outcomes that are both rational and efficient. In other words, our goal is to choose a set of welfare weights and then mathematically identify policies and allocations of resources that maximize the social welfare function (SWF):

$$\text{SWF} \equiv \sum_{i=1}^{N} \theta_i E[U(C_i)W(H_i)] \qquad (12.1a)$$

subject to any relevant social resource constraints. From an economic viewpoint, interventions are welfare-improving if they increase this measure of social welfare.

Consider an intervention that changes consumption and health from (C_i^0, H_i^0) to (C_i^T, H_i^T) and produces the change in total expected utility, ΔEU^T. Harsanyi's (1955) framework would measure the social value from introducing any treatment, T, in utility terms as

$$\Delta \text{SWF} \equiv \sum_{i=1}^{N} \theta_i \Delta EU^T \qquad (12.1b)$$

The more that social welfare goes up, the more valuable the intervention, and vice versa. Note that this focuses on *changes* in social welfare attributable to a medical innovation, not the *levels* of social welfare preceding the introduction of technology *T*. In this way, for example, this approach does not explicitly seek to correct existing disparities in income or health status unless these personal attributes enter into the determination of the θ_i weights.

THE WELFARE APPROACH OF TRADITIONAL CEA

These preliminaries raise two questions about welfare analysis of medical technologies. First, does cost-effectiveness analysis lead to sound and rigorous conclusions about social welfare? In other words, does CEA maximize a weighted sum of expected utilities, for some set of weights? It turns out the answer is "yes." This is good news because it justifies the use of CEA for analysis of welfare. However, the second question is trickier: What weights does traditional cost-effectiveness use, and do those weights seem ethically justified? Here, the news is less good, as we will see.

At least since the pioneering work of Philipson and Jena (2006) on the social value of HIV treatments, economists have measured the social value of new medical technologies by adding up the net monetary benefit to patients. Under conventional CEA and a Kaldor–Hicks view of welfare, this consists of value from the associated gain in quality-adjusted life years (QALYs), less any costs, and plus any relevant cost offsets. QALY gains are valued at K per QALY. To fix ideas, define CNMB_i^T as the "conventional net monetary benefit" accruing to individual i from technology T under "conventional" CEA. Social value under conventional CEA consists of

$$\mathrm{CNMB}^T \equiv \sum_{i=1}^{N} \mathrm{CNMB}_i^T \qquad (12.2a)$$

A key insight here is that the net monetary benefit for a particular patient is proportional to the change in monetized utility that results from introducing the technology, where

$$\mathrm{CNMB}_i^T = \frac{\Delta EU_i^T}{U'(C_{i0})W(H_{i0})} \qquad (12.2b)$$

The net monetary benefit of the new technology is the change in expected utility scaled by the marginal utility of consumption in the healthy, period 0 state, $U'(C_{i0})W(H_{i0})$. Intuitively, the marginal utility is the change in utility associated with one additional unit of consumption. This scaling converts from utility units to consumption units and yields a net monetary benefit expression. This is the same sort of "scaling" of utility as we introduced in Chapter 2.

In conventional CEA, $H_{i0} = 1$ because it assumes perfect health in the baseline state. Assuming without loss of generality that $W(1) = 1$, social value under traditional CEA is therefore given by

$$\text{CNMB} \equiv \sum_{i=1}^{N} \frac{\Delta \text{EU}_i^{\text{T}}}{U'(C_{i0})} \qquad (12.3)$$

Notice that this maps cleanly into the Harsanyi framework (Eq. 12.1b), provided that we define $\theta_i \equiv \dfrac{1}{U'(C_{i0})}$.

The good news is that the mapping to Harsanyi demonstrates that traditional CEA produces rigorous implications for welfare analysis. This reinforces the arguments of Garber and Phelps (1997). The bad news is that because of declining marginal utility of consumption, traditional CEA places more weight on people with higher levels of baseline consumption. In this situation, when $C_{i0} > C_{j0}$ and everybody is presumed to have the same utility function, then $U'(C_{i0}) < U'(C_{j0})$, which in turn implies that $\theta_i > \theta_j$.

Furthermore, even holding consumption fixed, people who are sicker at baseline receive the same utility weight as those who are healthier at baseline. Therefore, despite its provable rigor, traditional CEA embeds two distinct and unfavorable value judgments: Richer people get more weight than poorer people, and healthier people are given the same utility weight as sicker people. Things get even worse for sicker people if we also consider the fact that traditional CEA may understate their true gain in utility from treatment T, by ignoring diminishing returns to health. This also ignores the common empirical finding that income and health status are closely linked so that poorer people are also sicker people, on average.

A partial remedy to the problematic value judgments would be to equalize baseline levels of consumption. In other words, imagine that we treat everyone as if they have equal levels of baseline consumption. Many practitioners routinely employ this assumption by ignoring the actual distribution of wealth in the patient population and assuming that everyone enjoys the average per capita level of consumption prevailing in society. With this assumption in place, conventional CEA can get to equal utility weights, $\theta_i = \theta_j$, for all i, j. Gains in utility are treated as equal in value for all people.

This approach would not exacerbate inequality, but it does nothing to address it either. For instance, a sicker person who starts out at a lower level of utility does not receive any advantages over a healthier person who starts out with more utility. To make the example more concrete, suppose that there are equal numbers of sick and healthy people in society, where sick people enjoy utility of 10 "utils" and healthy people derive 20 utils. Imagine two new medical technologies: One provides 2 utils to all people, regardless of their health status. The other provides 4 utils to the sick and nothing to the healthy. Conventional CEA regards these two technologies as equal in Harsanyi's (1955) social welfare sense, even though the latter technology compresses inequality in health. Even this assessment is a bit too optimistic because conventional CEA systematically understates the gain in utility for sick patients relative to healthy patients. This is a question of accuracy, rather than of utility weights, but it nonetheless exacerbates inequality in practice. The following section describes how GRACE repairs this apparent inequity.

GRACE'S APPROACH TO WELFARE AND INEQUALITY

Does GRACE do any better than conventional CEA? We have already noted that GRACE gives sicker people their due when it comes to measuring the gains in utility that they derive from new medical technologies. This occurs because GRACE (through the R multiplier) properly expresses how the value of treatment increases as untreated illness severity rises. This compresses inequality relative to conventional CEA, even before considering how disability might affect the social welfare function (SWF) weights.

GRACE adds more than this when we consider its approach to incorporating permanent disability. Define GNMB_i^T as the "GRACE net monetary benefit" accruing to individual i from technology T under GRACE. Social value under GRACE consists of

$$\text{GNMB} \equiv \sum_{i=1}^{N} \text{GNMB}_i^T$$

As before, net monetary benefit for a particular patient is proportional to the change in utility that results from the technology, but under GRACE's disability adjustment, the marginal utility of consumption is allowed to vary with baseline permanent disability, giving

$$\text{GNMB}_i^T = \frac{\Delta \text{EU}_i^T}{U'(C_{i0})W(H_0(1-d^*))} \tag{12.4a}$$

Therefore, social value under GRACE can be rewritten as

$$\text{GNMB}^T \equiv \sum_{i=1}^{N} \frac{\Delta \text{EU}_i^T}{U'(C_{i0})W(H_0(1-d^*))} \tag{12.4b}$$

Notice how this captures the sense of preexisting disability that exists in period 0. As we did with the previous CEA analysis, we "monetize" the expected utility gains by dividing by the marginal utility of consumption. Since disability reduces the marginal utility of consumption, the value of health gains rises. As above, we will equalize consumption so that everyone is assumed to consume the same C_0 in the baseline period. Thus, GRACE is equivalent to a Harsanyi social welfare function, where $\theta_i \equiv \dfrac{1}{U'(C_0)W(H_0(1-d^*))}$. Recall from Chapter 5 that $\dfrac{W(H_0(1-d^*))}{W(H_0)} = 1 - \psi d^*$. Therefore, continuing with our normalization that $W(H_0) = 1$, GRACE implies utility weights of $\theta_i = \dfrac{1}{U'(C_0)(1-\psi d^*)}$, equivalent to what we defined in Chapter 5 as the disability-based multiplier D. In terms of Harsanyi's SWF structure, it follows that $\theta_i = D_i$.

In this revised model, people who have lower baseline health from disability will receive higher utility weights, and vice versa. GRACE embeds a natural approach to compressing inequality across health status by placing more weight on the utility of people with disability. This is an attractive feature compared to the conventional CEA approach because it incorporates a preference for equity into the standard neo-classical social welfare framework that is otherwise agnostic about equity considerations.

WELFARIST VERSUS EXTRA-WELFARIST VALUATION

Contrasting Methods for Valuing Health Gains

Particularly in nations with centralized health care systems, a new method to measure value has emerged, commonly called "extra-welfarism" (EW). For further details on these issues, (see Phelps 2023). Welfarist economics (WE) methods, which include GRACE, rely wholly on individuals' preferences to measure value. Harsanyi's (1955) proof shows that the proper method to combine individual measures of value to a SWF is a weighted sum of expected utilities (see Eq. 12.1a).

In contrast, EW practitioners eschew use of individual welfare measures. In health systems with fixed budget constraints, they replace the utilities of individuals with measures of their health. Although this is not the only possible way to conduct EW analyses, it is by far the most common. In one review, Brouwer et al. (2008) state that "health has become seen as the central (if not exclusive) focus of evaluations [in EW]" (p. 332). Coast (2009) summarizes this literature review by stating that "in practice, and despite protestations that extra-welfarism is not limited to the evaluative space of health alone . . . the practical exposition of the extra-welfarist approach is (almost?) entirely limited to the evaluative space of health" (p. 786). We thus will assume that EW methods equate with using H as the maximand.

Adopting this meaning of EW, we will show that EW is simply a constrained form of WE, just as CEA is a constrained form of GRACE.

This conclusion will allow us to apply Harsanyi's (1955) approach to EW models of value. To see this, begin with our standard model of value for a representative consumer:

$$V_j(C_j, H_j) = U_j(C_j)W_j(H_j) \qquad (12.5a)$$

First, impose CEA's typical restriction that there are constant returns to health in producing utility. Recall that this restriction represents the essential difference between CEA and GRACE, which imposes no such condition. In CEA, $W(H_j) = H_j$ (Garber and Phelps, 1997), so

$$V_j(C_j, H_j) = U_j(C_j)H_j \qquad (12.5b)$$

Next, assume the restriction that health system budgets are fixed. In this case, for each representative individual, consumption is fixed since C_j equals income minus medical spending, which does not vary with alternative health care technology choices. Moreover, CEA practitioners often perform health technology assessments under the assumption of income and consumption equality. Failure to do so places more weight on the health gains of richer people and less on poorer people. We previously suggested the same approach for welfare analyses using GRACE. Thus, we assume that $C_j = C$ for all j members of the society. Without loss of generality, therefore, we can now define our representative consumer's utility of consumption as $U_j(C_j) = 1$. Then

$$V_J(C_j, H_j) = H_j \qquad (12.6)$$

After we impose CEA's restriction of constant returns to health improvement and uniform consumption, WE simply becomes maximization of health, which is precisely the same as EW.

Now, because we have shown that EW is a restricted form of WE, we can legitimately use Harsanyi's (1955) proof to define social welfare functions within the EW restrictions:

$$\text{SWF}_{\text{EW}} = \sum_j \theta_j H_j \qquad (12.7)$$

As we have noted, the weights do not come from economic theory but, rather, from other considerations, such as equity, social justice, health status, or even from pure political bargaining. If social decision-makers have concerns that the true normalization of $U_j(C_j) = 1$ does not represent societal values, they can offset that by altering the values of θ_j appropriately to incorporate value preferences relating to the distribution of income.

Recall from Chapter 2 that the marginal rate of substitution, which determines the WTP for health improvements, is given as

$$\text{MRS} = \frac{V'_H(C,H)}{V'_C(C,H)} = \frac{\left[W'(H)U(C)\right]}{\left[U'(C)W(H)\right]} \qquad (12.8a)$$

But since $W(H) = H$ and $W'(H) = 1$ in EW valuations,

$$\text{MRS}_{\text{EW}} = \frac{U(C)}{U'(C)}\left[\frac{1}{H}\right] = K^B \qquad (12.8b)$$

In fixed-budget systems, K^B is set administratively, defined implicitly by the budget. Consumption, C, is fixed at average income minus the taxes necessary to support the central health care system. K^B differs from the WE-based measure of K in standard CEA or K^D_{GRACE}, which introduce trade-offs between consumption and health. Individuals at different incomes may prefer different thresholds, but the system operates as if everybody has the same WTP threshold, K^B. The threshold K^B is defined by the consumption level C allowed after taxes to support the health care system are removed from income.

The EW approach cannot possibly incorporate any of the adjustments to K that GRACE creates—including the adjustment for diminishing returns to health, ω_H, the severity of illness adjustment R, and the disability adjustment factor D—nor the adjustment to account for variable treatment outcomes, ε. Instead, several European nations have turned to ad hoc methods to adjust WTP for illness severity using authors' statements of what constitutes "ethical" or "fair" weighting systems. Although we discussed these approaches briefly in Chapter 10, we extend that analysis here.

Severity Adjustments in Current Use

For further details on these issues, see (Phelps and Lakdawalla 2023).

BACKGROUND

Two major issues arise in these deliberations. First is whether health loss should be measured on an absolute or proportional basis. The second is whether only future health gains and losses matter, or whether previous illness events (or permanent disabilities) should also enter the prioritization methodology.

Figure 12.1 provides the basis for describing these approaches—absolute shortfall (AS) and proportional shortfall (PS). These approaches rely on standard CEA methods where the QALY is the method used to combine gains in LE and HRQoL and measure their value. Area A describes remaining QALYs for an untreated person, combining LE along the horizontal axis and HRQoL on the vertical axis. For a treatment that increases HRQoL but does not alter LE, the gain in QALYs is shown in Area B. For a treatment that adds LE but does not alter HRQoL, the gain

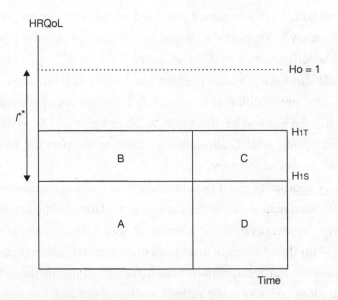

Figure 12.1 Panel A represents remaining QALYs for an untreated individual. Panel B shows HRQoL gains with no gain I LE. Panels C and D show QALY gains when the treatment extends LE and incorporates the gains in HRQoL in the extended period of LE.

is shown in Area D. Figure 12.1c shows the HRQoL gains associated with any LE gains. Treatments that improve LE and confer the same gains in HRQoL for the extended LE incorporate Area C as the final value gain.

In the United Kingdom, the National Institute for Health and Care Excellence (NICE) defines AS as "the total amount of future health they are expected to lose as a result of their condition." Specifically, AS is defined as $AS = B + C + D$. It shows the health loss that a person has from an untreated health condition relative to that of a person who receives the treatment. This approach directly flows from standard CEA methods for valuing gains and losses in health. PS is defined as $PS = \dfrac{AS}{A + B + C + D}$ (Towse and Barnsley, 2013).

Also discussed is the concept of "fair innings," which apparently relates to the games of cricket (in the United Kingdom and the British Commonwealth) and baseball (in East Asia and the Americas), wherein each team has an equal allotment of "innings" to attempt to score. In health care settings, it has been interpreted generally as the notion that every person is entitled to health care that will create a "normal" LE and HRQoL, but once that horizon has been reached, the priority for additional health care falls (described sometimes as "living on borrowed time"). This approach is widely viewed as discriminatory against older persons. In concept, it also places more value on treating persons who have lived a long time with a permanent disability, which has reduced the number of "fair innings" that they may have so far enjoyed. With this background, we next discuss several severity-adjustment systems in current use.

THE BRITISH NATIONAL HEALTH SERVICE AND NICE

The most recent NICE policy statement specifies direct adjustments for severity of illness based on either relative or absolute shortfall (see discussion below).[3] NICE's report provides its final severity modifier cutoffs and QALY weights as shown in Table 12.1. These criteria obviously add value only for the most severe diseases, with proportional shortfalls of 85% loss of HRQoL or more or absolute shortfalls of at least 12 QALYs. These choices are inconsistent with a full GRACE-based approach, but they do indicate that consideration of severity of illness has officially entered the NICE methodology.

Table 12.1 SEVERITY ADJUSTMENTS ADOPTED BY
NICE IN 2021

QALY Weight	Proportional QALY Shortfall	Absolute QALY Shortfall
1	<0.85	<12
×1.2	0.85–0.95	12–18
×1.7	≥0.95	≥18

THE NETHERLANDS

In the Netherland, the National Healthcare Institute (Zorginstitute Nederland [ZIN]) initially recommended (in 2006) a continuous severity/value curve with values ranging up to €80,000 per QALY, an upper bound with specific reference to the World Health Organization recommendation of 3X per capita gross domestic product as a maximum threshold, as discussed in Chapter 7. A decade after initial discussion about the concept, ZIN adopted a three-category threshold system as shown in Table 12.2. This system incorporates a fourfold increase in WTP for the highest severity conditions relative to lower severity conditions.

SWEDEN AND NORWAY

The concept of severity adjustment for WTP is common in Scandinavian nations (Barra et al., 2020), but the specific implementation methods remain under extensive discussion. Barra et al. conclude that "severity is poorly understood, and that the topic needs substantial further inquiry" (p. 25). For Norway, Ottersen et al. (2016) proposed a method in which

Table 12.2 THRESHOLDS PER QALY GAINED IN ZIN

Burden of Illness (Proportional Shortfall)	Maximum Threshold per QALY Gained
0.1–0.4	€20,000 (~$23,000)
0.41–0.7	€50,000 (~$56,000)
0.71–1.00	€80,000 (~$92,000)

Adapted from Reckers-Droog et al. (2018).

"the priority of an intervention increases with the expected lifetime health loss of the beneficiary in the absence of such an intervention" (p. 246). This "absolute shortfall" proposal addressed an ongoing debate in Norway about the proper method for measuring severity of illness.

Replacing earlier recommendations, the 2015 Magnussen report on severity[4] focused on differences arising from "absolute" and "proportional" shortfall methods that should receive higher priority. The Magnussen report concluded that "absolute shortfall incorporates to a greater degree than . . . other measures the key features of what characterizes a condition as severe."

The Magnussen report divides severity into six groups while stating that a continuous measure gives a false sense of accuracy. The lowest group consists of diseases/conditions for which the AS is less than 4 healthy life years, whereas the highest group includes conditions for which the expected absolute shortfall is more than 20 healthy life years. The report further proposed that the WTP for the lowest group be NOK 275,000 (~$30,000 per QALY) and NOK 825,000 for the highest severity group (~$90,000 per QALY). Therefore, the ratio between highest and lowest severity conditions is a factor of three.

Sweden's health system also features a grouped-by-severity WTP criterion (Barra et al., 2020). The highest degree of severity merits WTP values of 1,000,000 SEK (~$110,000) per QALY, 750,000 SEK (~$82,500) per QALY for "severe" conditions, 500,000 SEK (~$55,000) per QALY for conditions of a moderate degree, with a similar decrement for the lowest severity conditions (~$27,500 per QALY). The WTP ratio from lowest to highest severity is a factor of four, as in the Netherlands system. The Swedish system, in sharp contrast to the Norwegian system, has an absolute ban on valuation methods that incorporate chronological age, which precludes use of absolute shortfall measures.

Comparing Absolute Shortfall and Proportional Shortfall to GRACE

Both AS and PS diverge importantly from the concepts embedded in GRACE. We can best understand these by first examining how AS deals with increases in HRQoL (leaving LE unchanged). Here, AS conflates the *value per QALY* created by a treatment with the total QALYs created. AS assigns increasing value per QALY to interventions that have larger total gains in HRQoL. Holding baseline health constant, this is the reverse of what diminishing marginal utility of health indicates as the proper way to value interventions. In GRACE, diminishing returns specify that the value per QALY (expressed in the WTP formula $K_{GRACE} = K\omega_H R$) show that the value of larger QALY gains is less than linear, since $\omega_H < 1$. The only possible "saving grace" (pardon the pun) of the AS method is that very large gains can only be conferred upon those with poor initial HRQoL (hence having a high value of R). The proper solution, of course, is to focus directly on the initial untreated HRQoL, not the absolute magnitude of the QALY gain.

Absolute shortfall further diverges from standard economic analysis—both standard CEA and GRACE—by conferring increasing value per QALY to gains in LE. To see this, consider a treatment that makes no change in HRQoL but increases LE by, for example, more than 4 QALYs. The Norwegian system, as proposed by the Magnussen report, would increase the value per QALY for greater gains in LE, extending at high as a threefold multiplier for gains above 20 QALYs.

Standard CEA and the economic theory around the value of mortality reduction imply that people are risk neutral on this dimension of value, which means that they have constant returns to scale in QALY gains arising from LE gains. A 25% gain in LE leads to a 25% gain in value, *except for discounting*, which diminishes the value of incremental LE in a systematic (and well-known) way. Therefore, assigning greater value per QALY in the AS system to gains in LE reverses the effect of discounting. It is easy to envision situations in which the AS adjustment leads to de facto negative discount rates for gains in LE. The PS method contains the same errors as does AS because it simply normalizes AS in proportion to the potential maximum value of QALY increases. Therefore, the same criticisms apply to PS as to AS.

Finally, we comment on the fair innings concept, as discussed by Williams (1997), which looks backward in time to value future QALY gains. The concept is that a person who has suffered a long lifetime of QALY loss due to disability should place higher value on future QALY improvements. No other economic valuation model looks backward in time to consider previous life history as relevant to measuring future value.

To demonstrate the potential conflicts within this approach, consider two individuals, one of whom has been a paraplegic in a wheelchair for a lifetime and the other who has had normal health for the same life span. Now assume that the second individual has an accident that puts that person in the same situation as the first, namely confined to a wheelchair as a paraplegic. Finding a treatment that would improve the HRQoL for the second person would have low value in the fair innings approach because years of healthy life would weigh down the value measure. The first person would have a higher valuation for the same QALY improvement.

GRACE reaches a similar conclusion about valuation of future QALY improvements for these two hypothetical persons, but for a very different reason. GRACE states that preexisting disabilities lead to an adjustment in WTP of the magnitude D because of the diminished marginal utility of consumption associated with the lower HRQoL imposed by the disability. If anything, because of the absence of assimilative or adaptive coping by the newly injured person, GRACE would measure a higher value per QALY gain for the more recently injured individual.

Stairstep Methods

All current European severity adjustment methods use "stairstep" formulas to add value for treatment of increasingly high disease severity categories, commonly three or four levels [1, 2]. These typically range from multipliers of 1 (for least severe illnesses) to 4 (for most severe illnesses).

Two problems emerge from these stairstep approaches. First, stairsteps' widths and adjustment values are wholly arbitrary, as the large differences across current applications of these concepts demonstrate. Also, stairstep methods of assigning value fail on important equity grounds (Skedgel et al., 2022).

To understand these concerns, see Figure 12.2, which shows typical stairstep multipliers. Three different possible GRACE severity adjustment multiplier curves are shown, R_1, R_2, and R_3. R_2 is designed to pass through the middle of each stairstep. If R_2 is the correct R curve, then each stairstep has the proper valuation at least at its midpoint, but if other R curves are correct, the stairsteps misstate the proper value multiplier, perhaps everywhere.

There could be other R curves. These are arbitrary examples, unknown until the degree of risk aversion in HRQoL is measured. If risk aversion is "high," then R_3 is more likely to be correct, and conversely for R_1. Once the necessary risk parameters are estimated, GRACE provides methodologically based continuous severity adjustment methods, contrasting with arbitrary stairstep methods.

In addition, for wide illness severity ranges within any single stairstep, vertical equity is violated because people in different circumstances

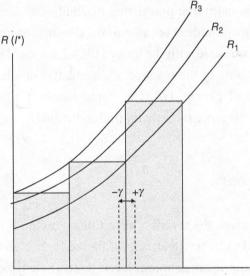

Figure 12.2 The horizontal axis represents illness severity, e.g, losses in HRQoL. The vertical axis indicates the illness severity measure R as defined in GRACE. The three gray bars represent typical "stair-step" adjustments in WTP for different levels of illness severity. The three curves represent possible severity-index curves that GRACE might lead to, depending on the degree of risk aversion in health. The main text discusses their interpretation. The dotted lines indicate possible small differences in patients' illness severity near the boundary between two stair-steps. The main text describes their interpretation.

(different severity levels) are treated identically. Only narrowing each stairstep's width can solve this problem, which asymptotically leads to continuous severity measures.

Measurement errors in severity levels can also worsen horizontal equity. Consider two patients with severity levels differing from any stairstep boundary by a small amount, γ, as shown in Figure 12.2. The first would have lower multiplier than the second, even though only small difference in AS or PS separate them. This violates horizontal equity, which states that people in similar circumstances should be treated similarly.

UTILITY MAXIMIZATION WITHIN FIXED-BUDGET SYSTEMS USING EXTRA-WELFARISM

Development of EW methods to value health care often comes in parallel with evaluation of health care systems that operate with fixed budgets. As discussed previously, this approach replaces $W(H)$ with H. We next address the question of how to incorporate the effects of fixed budgets in assessing the total value of health produced within the system.

We can analyze fixed-budget health systems as having two inputs, a and b. The fixed budget for the health system is $B = p_a a + p_b b$, so $\Delta b = -\dfrac{p_a}{p_b}\Delta a$. Each expanded use of a requires a reduction in input b, the amount determined by their relative costs to the health system. Proponents of EW methods call this the health opportunity cost of expanding the use of an intervention—that is, reduced health arising from the reduction in input b. In standard WE, the opportunity cost of improved health is reduced consumption.

To be clear, the trade-off between consumption and health sits at the center of WE methods to value health improvement, the "consumption" opportunity cost. By limiting the budget to a fixed level, EW can reduce overall welfare as measured by WE—that is, $V(H,C) = U(C)W(H)$.

How is aggregate welfare improvement measured in this system? Define H_a' and H_b' as the marginal health gains from increasing inputs a and b. The cost-effectiveness ratios of inputs a and b are defined as $\text{CE}_a = \dfrac{p_a}{H_a'}$ and $\text{CE}_b = \dfrac{p_b}{H_b'}$. Now

$$\Delta H = H_a'\Delta a + H_b'\Delta b = \Delta a\frac{p_a}{\text{CE}_a} - \Delta a\left[\frac{p_a}{p_b}\right]\left[\frac{p_b}{\text{CE}_b}\right] \qquad (12.9a)$$

Simplifying Equation (12.9a) and defining the "displacement effect" factor as $\text{DE} \equiv \left[\dfrac{\left[\text{CE}_b - \text{CE}_a\right]}{\text{CE}_a\text{CE}_b}\right]$, we now have

$$\Delta H = p_a\Delta a\left[\frac{1}{\text{CE}_a} - \frac{1}{\text{CE}_b}\right] = p_a\Delta a\left[\frac{\left[\text{CE}_b - \text{CE}_a\right]}{\text{CE}_a E_b}\right] = p_a\Delta a\text{DE} \qquad (12.9b)$$

This proves that $\dfrac{\Delta H}{\Delta a} > 0$ if and only if $\text{CE}_b > \text{CE}_a$. In words, this simply means that input b is less cost-effective than input a. This well-known result shows why practitioners of EW commonly focus on incremental cost-effectiveness ratios to assess changes in a health system's operation. To improve health, and hence the restricted form of utility, health care systems must increase the use of inputs with lower CE ratios and decrease the use of those with higher CE ratios. In equilibrium, if all inputs can be adjusted continuously, every input (treatment) has the same incremental CE ratio, equal to K^B, as implicitly defined by the budget constraint. Of course, lumpiness in technologies makes this exact equilibrium infeasible.

With this background, consider now the issue of weighted societal preferences. Using the EW approach, the Harsanyi-based SWF is

$$\text{SWF}_{\text{EW}} = \sum_i \theta_i H_i \qquad (12.10a)$$

so that

$$\Delta SWF_{EW} = \sum_i \theta_i \Delta H_i \qquad (12.10b)$$

Changes in the SWF must assess the effect of changes in each H_i. If every member of society receives an equal weight—for example, $\theta_j = \dfrac{1}{N}$ in a society of N individuals—then the standard CEA methods of evaluation apply. Only the aggregate change in health matters. This, we believe, has been the primary focus of most EW technology evaluations to date.

However, if different individuals have different weights in the SWF, then one must consider the impact on each member of society by changing the allocation of the fixed budget between inputs a and b. Health technology assessment methods must now evaluate this expression for each consumer enrolled in the health care system:

$$\Delta H_i = H_a' \Delta a_i + H_b' \Delta b_i \qquad (12.10c)$$

If different individuals differentially use inputs a or b, then this evaluation must assess individual changes in utilization, Δa_i and Δb_i, and their aggregate effect, ΔH_i. The aggregate budget constraint results may not accurately portray the effects of a technology change on individuals or subpopulations.

Health technology evaluation must now consider the differential effects of policy changes on individuals or subpopulations of interest and then aggregate those effects using the weights in the SWF. This complicates the problem of maximizing expected utility (health) in fixed-budget systems. No longer does the aggregate displacement effect DE determine changes in the SWF. Indeed, the problem gets even worse if H_a' or H_b' vary by subpopulation, as is true for some medical interventions.

To be clear, the same complexity exists using the GRACE-based SWF shown in Eq. (12.4b). That SWF adds up the changes in health for each individual, adjusted by the weight D_i, the value adjustment arising from preexisting disability.

To provide a simple example, suppose that input a represented Pap smears to detect cervical cancer in women and input b represented prostate-specific antigen (PSA) tests to detect prostate cancer in men. Then increasing the use of Pap smear tests on the extensive margin (recommended age brackets for testing) or the intensive margin (recommended frequency of testing) would require reductions in PSA along one or both margins. If women's health were rated differently than men's health, simple measures of the aggregate change in H would not suffice to determine the change in the SWF in Eq. (12.10b).

Suppose, similarly, that a subpopulation was identified that had predictably low levels of health for various reasons, such as income, racial bias, or urban/rural status. Societal preferences toward equalizing health outcomes of all individuals would lead to shifting resources toward treatment or other interventions that specifically improved the health of that subpopulation, even though it would come at the expense of reducing the health of the broader population because of the fixed-budget constraint. This would lead to a convergence in achieved health outcomes both by increasing the health of those with the poorest baseline health and by decreasing health for those with higher levels of baseline health.

Some methods of technology evaluation, such as expanded CEA (Vergout et al., 2016) or the broader "augmented CEA" (Lakdawalla et al., 2018), measure the effects of interventions on various subpopulations but do not provide methods for determining the weights on the health of each identified subpopulation. We believe that the best methods for determining weights to combine them will focus on deliberative processes, preferably augmented using multi-criteria decision analysis (MCDA) techniques (Phelps and Madhavan, 2017, 2021; Phelps et al., 2018). Among other benefits of this approach, it provides higher levels of transparency to the public about how the societal preference weights are determined.

SUMMARY

Comparatively little attention has been paid to the underlying implications of conventional cost-effectiveness for inequality. In this chapter, we show that the conventional approach suffers from several undesirable features: It fails to account for the proper gain in utility that sick patients derive from medical technology; and it employs equal utility weights for people with both poor and good baseline health. GRACE, on the other hand, places more utility weight on those with greater baseline disability, promoting equality of expected utility.

However, there are aspects of inequality that GRACE does not address, principally those involving externalities in health care, such as scientific spillovers, value of health improvement to patients' family members, and the like. The analysis in this chapter presents a path forward for incorporating these. Beginning with net monetary benefit measures of these quantities, we can convert these into expected utility gains and exploit the existing neoclassical framework for evaluating inequality. Some considerations involving the distribution of income emerge in the specific issue of how consumption income, C, might affect utility weights and whether the analyst should attempt to mitigate these effects.

In terms of equity, GRACE only informs the discussion in two specific dimensions of equity that are commonly considered—severity of illness and degree of permanent disability. Many other dimensions of equity appear on the societal agenda, including those involving race, ethnicity, sexual orientation, nationality of origin, geographic location, access to care, degree of insurance coverage, and others. However, a wide literature shows that degrees of illness severity and disability are strongly correlated to some of these measures, most notably race, income, ethnicity, and (less well-documented) sexual orientation. Therefore, improvement in the social contract regarding illness and disability severity could, through the established correlations, improve equity at least partially on some of these other dimensions of equity.

With regard to consideration of scientific spillover as well as the multiplicity of issues involving equity and fairness, improving public policy will almost certainly require invoking other approaches to establishing the relative magnitude of importance on these other dimensions of value. One widely cited methodology is MCDA, which provides formal methods to assess relative value of different aspects of medical interventions (Phelps and Madhavan, 2017, 2021; Phelps et al., 2018). Elaboration of these issues extends beyond the scope of this book.

Furthermore, current EW methods fail to deal with illness severity and disability in coherent ways. Major differences in ethical and fairness dimensions appear between AS and PS. It is not possible for both these methods to be correct, because they diverge so markedly. Despite that divergence, both AS and PS methods are in current use in European nations. The most striking example occurs in the current NICE methods for severity adjustment, which calculate adjustments for any specific technology using both AS and PS and then accept the greater of the two adjustments that emerge from the analysis. In effect, this indicates that the decision-makers do not know which is correct (if either), so they satisfy proponents of both methods by using the highest score from each method. This "political" solution has no apparent basis in economics, ethics, philosophy, or other notions of fairness.

Similarly, the divergence between Norway's use of AS and Sweden's outright rejection of AS in favor of PS shows that no clear basis exists for choosing between these two adjustment methods. In related writings and rhetoric, the concept of age bias looms large for opponents of AS, and this concern arises also in the fair innings approach.

Conclusions and Next Steps

The secret of getting ahead is getting started.

—Mark Twain

SUMMARY OF ISSUES

The generalized risk-adjusted cost-effectiveness (GRACE) model begins with traditional cost-effectiveness analysis (CEA) as first formalized by Garber and Phelps (1997) and generalizes it with one simple change: It introduces diminishing returns to HRQoL instead of assuming constant returns, the position built into traditional CEA.

That one simple change has profound implications for the proper practice of CEA, ranging from the way a quality-adjusted life year (QALY) is valued to how many "equivalent" QALYs are created by treatments with uncertain health outcomes. Perhaps most radically, it turns upside down the normal CEA model, which states that improving the health or longevity of disabled people has less value than providing the same improvement for otherwise-similar nondisabled persons.

Valuing Health. Charles E. Phelps and Darius N. Lakdawalla, Oxford University Press. © Oxford University Press 2024.
DOI: 10.1093/oso/9780197686287.003.0013

The GRACE method produces five major changes in the proper method to carry out technology valuations that previously would have used CEA methods:

1. Because of diminishing returns to H, the basic willingness to pay (WTP) value declines, compared with the traditional CEA model. Where the elasticity of utility with respect to H is ω_H, the basic WTP measure is the traditional measure $\left(K = \dfrac{C}{\omega_C} \right)$ multiplied by ω_H. If $\omega_H = 0.5$, for example, then the basic WTP in traditional CEA is twice as large as GRACE indicates that it should be.

2. Offsetting that decline in the base level WTP, GRACE states that there should be a severity adjustment (R) increasing WTP as untreated illness severity increases. Chapter 2 discusses these adjustments in detail, and Chapters 9 and 11 give further examples of the interactions between ω_H and r_H^* in determining the final value measure, K_{GRACE}.

3. The traditional model ignores variability in treatment outcomes. However, when people have declining marginal utility in H, they are also risk averse in health, the extent to which this occurs being summarized in the risk aversion parameter r_H^*, expanded to provide more precision by including relative prudence (π_H^*) and possibly even relative temperance (τ_H^*). Chapter 3 discusses these issues and provides specific methods to measure the value-changing effects of uncertain treatment outcomes.

4. When considering the trade-off between LE and HRQoL, formally, the marginal rate of substitution (MRS), the traditional model, by assuming constant returns to health also assumes that the MRS is constant across all levels of HRQoL. Introducing diminishing returns to health demonstrates why this MRS should vary as base-level HRQoL differs from situation to situation. We provide methods to estimate this parameter in Chapter 4.

5. The proper consideration of permanent disability is flipped on its head compared with traditional CEA methods. The mathematics of the traditional CEA model clearly specify that improving the health or longevity of a disabled person is worth less than doing so an otherwise-similar nondisabled person. In our notation herein, this is the distinction between K_{GRACE} and K_{GRACE}^{D}. Instead, GRACE unambiguously shows that improving HRQoL for permanently disabled people has higher, not lower, value than for a comparable nondisabled person. Further adjustments to the model, discussed in Chapter 5, add to the value of improving HRQoL for disabled people, although there remains some ambiguity about the net effect on LE extensions in some situations because of conflicting factors in the overall GRACE method. We believe that further research may show that these situations are either rare or (in some cases) do not exist.

With these "pieces" in place, Chapter 6 extends the analysis to multi-period models, Chapter 7 provides methods to estimate cost-effectiveness thresholds, Chapter 8 explains how to estimate GRACE's relative risk parameters, and Chapter 9 summarizes this work with examples of each type of necessary calculation. Chapters 10 and 11 explore transition issues and consequences of health plans' adoption of GRACE. Chapter 12, which contains an entirely new direction of analysis within the GRACE context, explores ethical issues arising from use of standard CEA and shows how GRACE eliminates or counteracts these problems.

IMPLEMENTATION OF GRACE

GRACE is more difficult to implement than traditional CEA. In the most general case, it requires new information about people's attitudes toward risky health outcomes and about the rate at which utility of H declines as H improves (ω_H is the key parameter). A simpler method arises if analysts are willing to assume a specific form of the utility function $W(H)$ with appropriately estimated parameters. Functions in common use elsewhere in the economics literature include constant relative risk aversion and hyperbolic absolute risk aversion (HARA) utility, as discussed in previous chapters, and expo-power utility (Saha, 1993).[1]

GRACE also requires new measures of variance and skewness of the treatment outcomes for each medical intervention under evaluation, in addition to parallel measures for the "comparison" treatment that CEA and GRACE require.[2] Fortunately, the underlying data for all of these measures already exist in the "raw" data compiled in typical health outcomes studies such as randomized controlled trials and comparative effectiveness studies.

The new preference parameter estimates need not be undertaken by every health technology assessment (HTA). Once these parameters have been estimated a number of times by professionals accomplished in the necessary methodologies, a consensus should develop around the proper parameter values for $\omega_H, r_H^*, \pi_H^*, \tau_H^*$ and an understanding of how these may or may not vary across different levels of health.

This implementation task can be even simpler when using the exact utility function approach. Standard methods to estimate risk aversion, particularly discrete choice experiments (DCEs) assume a specific utility function, so when the relevant parameters are estimated, applying the exact utility function for $W(H)$ is straightforward. Appendix 6.1 provides pertinent details. Because traditional HTA studies will almost always capture the necessary data to measure the variance, skewness, and perhaps the kurtosis measures required for GRACE, there is relatively little burden created for the proper conduct of HTA when using GRACE rather than traditional CEA methods. To us, "it's too hard" or "it requires too much new data" are not meaningful reasons for not adopting GRACE as the primary method for valuing medical interventions.

Numerous examples exist in which improvement in our understanding of the world around us required adopting more complicated mathematics. Without Kepler's understanding of elliptical (rather than circular) planetary orbits, we never would have mastered an understanding of how planets behave in their orbits. Ellipses are more difficult to compute than circles.

Similarly, major portions of modern society depend on electronic devices that use transistors. The behavior of electrons in solids cannot be understood without using quantum mechanics, so understanding how transistors work requires a level of mathematics far more complicated than the mathematics required to understand Newtonian mechanics.

Branches of mathematics that were once considered obscure and of no practical value continue to make their way into modern society. The field of algebraic topology, for example, provides the basis for reconstructing magnetic resonance imaging and computed tomography images from the amassed numerical data measured by these scanning instruments. Number theory has led to important advances in cryptology, device authentication, e-commerce, and security systems. These branches of mathematics are "hard" by almost any standard, but they also create valuable "things" that are unobtainable without the underlying math.

If cosmologists (in the first example), electrical engineers and computer scientists (in the second), medical device manufacturers (in the third), and internet developers (in the fourth example) had simply said, "The math is too hard," we never would have enjoyed the results of these inventions and ideas.

In GRACE, the increase in mathematical requirements is actually quite modest, involving (at a maximum) introductory calculus instead of the introductory algebra required for standard CEA. The additional computations to conduct GRACE analyses (compared with standard CEA) can readily be accomplished with simple spreadsheet software.

Moreover, in this book, we have outlined a number of approaches that reduce the empirical estimation requirements of GRACE—for example, the use of HARA utility to infer the entire set of risk preferences from just two parameters evaluated at any single health level and the computational methods to incorporate higher order risk preferences into the Taylor series expansions upon which rely (to estimate R, ψ, ρ, and ε). We have also provided algorithms that could be embedded in software tools that facilitate the conduct of GRACE analyses. In principle, analysts should be able to compute GRACE valuations based solely on (1) mean, variance, and skewness of HRQoL benefits, possibly varying over time; (2) mean longevity benefits; (3) relative risk aversion (r_H^*) and relative prudence (π_H^*); and (4) the HRQoL loss from disability (d^*), pretreatment illness (ℓ^*), and post-treatment illness (t^*). All the other methods of GRACE could be embedded into software tools for practitioners.

We again remind readers that the exact utility function approach further simplifies estimation of GRACE models. This approach bypasses the Taylor Series approximation processes for the key GRACE parameters. This may be particularly useful where illness severity levels are high, a situation in which Taylor series approximations may not converge rapidly.

REAL-WORLD IMPLEMENTATION OF GRACE

Nobody . . . repeat . . . nobody will instantly adopt GRACE as the method for valuing medical interventions. Setting aside from the "mere" problem of gaining agreement about the proper values for value parameters such as ω_H, r_H^*, and higher order risk parameters, a shift to GRACE-based valuations would require major re-evaluation of existing therapeutic alternatives in current use within a health care system (or as approved treatments within an insurance plan). That will not happen "soon," and probably not even in the intermediate term. This is a question of long-term integration of a new idea into functioning (and, it is hoped, learning) health care systems.

Several basic notions will likely drive the patterns of changeover from using no formal evaluation methods or standard CEA to GRACE:

1. The difference between GRACE and standard CE is not large for low-severity illnesses. Health plans seeking to migrate their evaluation methods to include GRACE should focus on treatments for the most severe illnesses, leaving treatments for less severe disorders and diseases for "mopping up."

2. Among higher severity illnesses, the highest priority should focus on evaluating treatments that are in relatively common use rather than treatments for rare diseases. This is simply a pragmatic observation that rare events do not affect average overall value very much (and hence only small effects on premiums, to the extent that new valuation methods carry into provider payments that in turn affect premiums). However, "rare diseases," although individually uncommon, can add up to important parts of health system budgets. Perhaps the most telling on this front is that 31 of 53 new-molecule-entity drug patents in 2020 (58 percent) came under the umbrella of the U.S. Food and Drug Administration's "orphan drug" procedures for rare diseases.[3]

3. The combination of these two concepts suggests an informal strategy for carrying out full GRACE technology value evaluations: (a) Conduct an inventory of treatments (or payments) that measures frequency and cost; (b) using such resources as the Tufts registry, create a preliminary list of disease severity associated with each high-cost, high-frequency treatment; and (c) create an index of severity × frequency × average cost. Procedures with a high index are ripe candidates for a full GRACE evaluation and comparison (where available) with alternative therapies.

Naturally, we believe that evaluations of new technologies should use GRACE wherever possible. Even before estimates of the key risk/utility parameters are developed, any agency using standard CEA can (and we believe should) begin to require statistical data necessary to carry out GRACE evaluations. With such data, once risk/preference parameters are developed, evaluative agencies can work backward to produce GRACE-based estimates of technology values. The key data from technology developers (biopharmaceutical, medical device, or medical procedures and strategies) already exist in standard clinical studies, so it is just a question of reporting these data along with currently required average data on outcomes, side effects, and adverse events. GRACE employs variances, measures of skewness, and (if possible) measures of kurtosis in the distribution of treatment outcomes in addition to the traditionally used mean values. These additional data are readily derived from the data already collected in standard clinical trials, comparative effectiveness studies, and related data-gathering efforts.

ECONOMIC EFFICIENCY AND EQUITY ISSUES

Economic Efficiency

To the extent that people's true preferences contain significant degrees of diminishing marginal utility and risk aversion in H, continuing to evaluate medical interventions using standard CEA methods creates socially inefficient choices compared with using GRACE methods to measure value. CEA was originally introduced to improve efficiency in settings in which market prices are distorted or absent, and in which CEA could serve as a proxy for market-based values. Extending that same logic, GRACE further increases societal efficiency by incorporating people's true attitudes toward uncertain treatment outcomes and how severity of illness properly factors into value measures.

Equity Considerations Regarding Disabled Individuals

Standard CEA methods contain mathematically based biases against disabled people. These biases have resulted in U.S. law banning the use of any CEA method that discounts the value of a life for a disabled person. comes specifically from the U.S. Affordable Care Act. Section 1182, 42 U.S.C. 1320e–1(c(1)) reads: "The Patient-Centered Outcomes Research Institute established under section 1181(b)(1) shall not develop or employ a dollars-per-quality adjusted life year (or similar measure that discounts the value of a life because of an individual's disability) as a threshold to establish what type of health care is cost effective or recommended. The Secretary shall not utilize such an adjusted life year (or such a similar measure) as a threshold to determine coverage, reimbursement, or incentive programs under title XVIII."

Several methods have attempted to "fix" this problem (Nord et al., 1999; Basu et al., 2020) by altering the QALYs assigned to disabled persons in HTA, thus reverting to counterfactual situations to resolve the problem.

Alternatively, GRACE recognizes the health status consequences of permanent disability, but it shows that the *value* assigned to treating disabled persons is greater (not less) than that for similar nondisabled persons. This eliminates the issue about methods "discounting" the value of a life because a person is disabled. We consider the current CEA method of valuing the health of disabled people to be not only mathematically wrong but also morally objectionable.

Other Equity Issues

GRACE is built upon the preferences of a rational, utility-maximizing individual. As such, it is an inadequate instrument to assess societal values that go beyond individual utility-maximizing valuations. The field of economics clearly recognizes this with regard to any "externality" and to considerations of the distribution of income or wealth, racial or other disparities in health, or differential access to health services.

The ISPOR "value flower" contains a number of "petals" that have previously been considered as beyond the ken of CEA and therefore requiring some additional analysis or consideration in terms of the overall value of a medical intervention or invention. Multi-criteria decision analysis provides one such tool (Phelps and Madhavan, 2017; Phelps et al., 2018).

By introducing non-constant returns to health, GRACE captures and enfolds in a coherent economic model four of these petals—insurance value, value of hope, severity of illness, and reduction in uncertainty. We believe that GRACE can help illuminate several other of these petals, although we have not attempted to incorporate these ideas herein. These include the "fear of contagion" and "real option value," the value of extending LE with the hope that a cure for an otherwise-fatal disease might be found during the added LE gained.

More generally, the ISPOR flower should be thought of not as a solution to what ails traditional CEA but, rather, as a list of symptoms that must be treated or cured. Critics have rightly pointed out that the petals of the flower might overlap, and it is inappropriate to compute each individual component of value and then add these up as an alternative approach to value assessment. What is needed is a single overarching framework that incorporates all the petals of the ISPOR flower and others that have yet to be identified. GRACE, we believe, represents a major step along the pathway to that goal.

FINAL THOUGHTS

Summarizing all of this, the current HTA model, based on standard CEA methodology, boldly and regularly asserts that "a QALY is a QALY is a QALY." GRACE demonstrates that this is not true when people have diminishing returns to health. From this come a number of important changes for the conduct of HTA: The underlying disability status of a person *does* matter when thinking about the value of QALYs. The untreated health status of an individual similarly matters, and a QALY of health gain to a person with very low untreated health is worth considerably more than a QALY of health gain to a person with mild illness. Separately, not all treatments with equal average outcomes are equivalent; they produce different levels of QALYs to people who have risk aversion in H.

These issues, we believe, provide the fundamental basis for HTAs and decision-makers using HTA models to shift to GRACE-based systems of value rather than continuing to use traditional CEA methods that do not capture peoples' true preferences about their level of health and uncertainty surrounding it.

APPENDIX 2.1

Previous Analyses Dealing with Diminishing
Returns/Uncertainty in Cost-Effectiveness Analysis

Unsurprisingly, we are not the first scholars to consider uncertainty in cost-effectiveness. Here, we summarize some of the earlier analyses, seeking to demonstrate where the field had come to as the point at which we began our work. We know of three studies, which we summarize briefly here in order of publication:

1. Joshua Graff-Zivin (2001) approached the problem by assuming stochastic effectiveness and fixed costs. He adopted an exponential utility function, which has constant absolute risk aversion (CARA), and then showed (with assumed risk aversion parameters) that for two interventions that are "cost-effective" using standard CEA methods, only one is cost-effective after taking uncertainty of outcomes into account. This model used only variance to measure uncertainty. It does not provide methods to distinguish between gains in HRQoL or LE, nor does it consider the parallel consequences of diminishing returns to health that risk aversion implies, including that WTP rises as untreated health falls.

2. Eliam Elbasha (2005) approached the problem by using an exponential utility function to describe a social planner's risk attitudes, where risk attitudes of each member of the society are

considered to be exponential (CARA utility). Elbasha used a moment-generating function approach to characterize the risk, of which the standard mean/variance approach is a subset. He assumes that the WTP parameter (π in his notation, K in ours) is known and fixed, and he uses that to create a net monetary benefit in the usual fashion. Where e_j is the incremental effectiveness of health program j, presumably measured in QALYs or some similar metric, and C_j is incremental cost, he denotes net benefit of intervention j as $NB_J = \pi e_j - c_j$. He then uses standard welfare economics approaches by expressing net welfare gain as a linear aggregation of individual utilities. The WTP parameter π monetizes health benefits. He then assumes a bivariate normal distribution of costs and effectiveness, thereby eliminating any issues associated with skewed or leptokurtic distributions of benefits or costs.

This approach intrinsically assumes that the same WTP exists for all levels of illness severity, thereby ignoring the diminishing returns to health outcomes that necessarily arise with risk aversion in health. It also automatically assumes that risk aversion in health and consumption are essentially identical, by first monetizing health outcomes and then applying the same risk parameter to both cost and health outcomes. This approach also does not specify how to combine improvements in HRQoL and LE, assuming instead that a combined measure "e" has been obtained.

3. Al et al. (2005) assumed decreasing value for both money and health effects, and they (along with others) assumed exponential utility to develop their mathematical presentation, using "consumption spending" (income minus medical expenses) as the appropriate measure of "money." As with others, these authors assume that a combined effectiveness measure "e" has been determined for each program being evaluated. There are no methods specifying for combining improvements to HRQoL and LE. Furthermore, their work does not pursue the consequences

of declining marginal utility of health that risk aversion in health requires. They provide a worked example in which utility is the sum of two exponential utility functions (again, with CARA utility), one for consumption and the other for health, each with their own risk parameters δ for consumption and γ for health outcomes, to demonstrate their method.

SUMMARY

All these earlier studies assessing risk in CEA have common features. By far the most important of these is that they overlook the consequences of diminishing returns to health that logically must exist if risk aversion exists. Therefore, they make no adjustment in the WTP measure to account for diminishing returns to health. In this sense, their work corresponds with the approach in Garber and Phelps (1997), who also assumed constant returns to health. The difference arises in the inconsistency: Garber and Phelps consistently assumed both constant marginal utility and no risk aversion, whereas these later studies inconsistently assumed risk aversion but constant marginal utility in health.

To put these issues into the notation we have adopted for GRACE, they have examined the implications of stochastic health outcomes that GRACE measures in ε while still maintaining that both ω_H and R equal 1.0. They all overlook the consequences of diminishing returns for health on the marginal rate of substitution between HRQoL and LE (because they all have a single "effect" measure that does not distinguish between HRQoL and LE gains). Furthermore, none of them assess the consequences of diminishing returns on the consequences for valuing health improvements for disabled persons.

These studies all adopted exponential utility as the desired functional form for utility, and they also limit their consideration of uncertainty to variances, thereby ignoring skewness (essential to our understanding of the value of hope) and kurtosis, which can also affect measures of value in GRACE.

Exponential utility has CARA, which is a very specific and probably unrealistic form of utility. CARA assumes that relative risk aversion increases linearly with income (or health). In the economics of finance and uncertainty, CARA has been widely rejected as an appropriate form for the utility function in money, and there is now reasonably widespread agreement that utility of money is reasonably well approximated by CRRA functions. The most flexible of these functions that we know of are HARA functions that we use in several places in this book.

To understand the problem associated with the use of CARA, consider the function for R, the severity of illness measure. In the Taylor series expansion, $R = 1 + \dfrac{r_H^* \ell^*}{1!} + \dfrac{1}{2!} r_H^* \pi_H^* \ell^{*2} + \dfrac{1}{3!} r_H^* \pi_H^* \tau_H^* \ell^{*3} + \ldots$

In CARA utility, $r_H^* = \pi_H^* = \tau^* = \ldots$. In CRRA utility, $\pi_H^* = r_H^* + 1, \tau_H^* = r_H^* + 2 \ldots$ and so forth. Thus, CARA undervalues higher order moments in the Taylor series expansion relative to CRRA utility. Of course, in studies that terminate the Taylor series at the variance term, this is not relevant because they wholly ignore skewness and kurtosis, rather than merely undervaluing them.

This affects the basic value multiplier because the proper starting point becomes not $K = \dfrac{C}{\omega_C}$ but, rather, $K = C \left[\dfrac{\omega_H}{\omega_C} \right]$, which in turn still misses the severity of illness multiplier R as well as key measures of the marginal rate of substitution between LE and HRQoL (ρ, used to estimate δ) and the key value ψ that affects the way disability affects value of health improvements, as discussed in Chapter 5.

Convergence of Taylor Series Estimates of R and Its Integral

As visual inspection of Eq. (2.9) reveals, the higher order terms become increasingly important as ℓ^* grows larger, and this is exacerbated for larger values of r_H^* and higher order risk preference terms. We begin this discussion with a method to provide an exact solution to one set of terms in Table 2.1, those arising when $r_H^* = 1$. In this case, with CRRA, then $\pi_H^* = 2, \tau_H^* = 3$.... etc. In this unique situation (across the bottom row of Table 2.1), as one can see from Eq. (2.9), the growing products of the risk parameters (e.g., r_H^*, π_H^*, τ_H^*) just offset the growing factorial powers in the denominator as specified by the Taylor series method. In this case, $R = \sum_{n=1}^{n} (\ell^*)^n$ and as n grows large, the series converges to the value of $\frac{1}{1-\ell^*}$. Thus, for example, when $\ell^* = 0.9$ in Table 2.1 for $r_H^* = 1$, $R = \frac{1}{0.1} = 10$. We can use this as a benchmark to assess the convergence of the Taylor series equation to estimate R.

For relatively large values of ℓ^* (i.e., values exceeding 0.8 or so), convergence is quite slow, requiring dozens of terms before the total converges to a fixed number to at least three decimal places. This is exacerbated at larger values of r_H^* (and successive risk terms) and reduced for lower values of r_H^*. At the extreme (the lower right-hand corner of Table 2.1), the actual Taylor series value at the 50th term was 9.93, not the value of 10 that we can calculate analytically (as in the previous paragraph). Convergence to two decimal places occurred at the 72nd term. At $\ell^* = 0.8$, convergence was achieved at 30 terms and at $\ell^* = 0.7$, 20 terms. At values of $\ell^* = 0.5$ and $r_H^* = 0.5$, convergence to three decimal places occurred at the fifth term. Thus, programmers should be sure to include a sufficient number of terms in the Taylor series expansions to achieve desired levels of convergence.

The Taylor series for the integral under the R curve (Eq. 2.11c) converges faster than the calculations for R itself. With the extreme values of $r_H^* = 1$ and $\ell^* = 0.9$, the Taylor series for the integral converges to two decimal places of accuracy at the 22rd term, whereas the calculation for R itself converges to that level of accuracy at the 72nd term. At lower levels of r_H^* and ℓ^*, the convergence rate is similar for both functions, and convergence occurs in just a few terms for smaller values of r_H^* and ℓ^*.

As Eq. (8.8) and the surrounding material in Chapter 8 demonstrate, a simple method exists to obtain these higher order risk parameters by adopting the HARA utility function. With the availability of HARA methods, we do not have concerns about slow convergence of the Taylor series terms because all higher order terms can be readily estimated by simply knowing two of the basic terms—for example, r_H^* and π_H^*. From these two estimates, τ_H^* and all higher order terms are instantly known.

Details in Measurement of ϵ

Technically, Eq. (3.1) also reflects the exclusion of other higher order terms involving squares, cubes, and fourth powers of the mean effects. A more extensive representation of ϵ, including these higher order terms, reads as

$$
\epsilon \equiv \left\{ 1 + \left[\frac{\mu_H}{\mu_B} \right] \left[\begin{array}{l} -\dfrac{1}{2} r_H^* \dfrac{[\Delta\sigma^2 + \mu_B^2]}{\mu_H^2} + \dfrac{1}{6} r_H^* \pi_H^* \dfrac{[\Delta\gamma\sigma^3 + 3\sigma_{H+B}^2 \mu_B + \mu_B^3]}{\mu_H^3} \\[2ex] -\dfrac{1}{24} r_H^* \pi_H^* \tau_H^* \dfrac{[\Delta\kappa + 6\sigma_{H+B}^2 \mu_B^2 + 4\mu_B \gamma\sigma_{H+B}^3 + \mu_B^4]}{\mu_H^4} + \cdots \end{array} \right] \right\}
$$

Notice that σ^2 is of the same order of magnitude as the squared mean, and $\gamma\sigma^3$ is of the order of the cubed mean. Thus, the excluded terms are of the magnitude equal to the squared mean or higher. Analysts are of course welcome to include them at their discretion, but in many real-world examples, they will be negligible.

We also note that these omitted terms have significant size only for relatively large values of μ_B (i.e., relatively large treatment effects). However, the leading term in the expression for ϵ, i.e., $\dfrac{\mu_H}{\mu_B}$, shows that the entire risk term has diminishing significance as μ_B rises. This further suggests that omission of these terms will have negligible effect in many real-world studies.

The same logic can be used to include the higher order terms in the formulation of Eq. (3.2c). In particular, all the higher order terms can be thought of as part of ε_T, as in

$$\varepsilon_T \approx \left[\frac{\mu_H}{\mu_B}\right]\left[\begin{array}{c} -\frac{1}{2}r_H^*\left(\frac{1}{\mu_H}\right)^2(\sigma_T^2 + \mu_B^2) + \frac{1}{6}\pi_H^* r_H^*\left(\frac{1}{\mu_H}\right)^3(\gamma_1^T\sigma_T^3 + +3\sigma_{H+B}^2\mu_B + \mu_B^3) \\ -\frac{1}{24}\tau_H^*\pi_H^* r_H^*\left(\frac{1}{\mu_H}\right)^4(\gamma_2^T\sigma_T^4 + 6\sigma_{H+B}^2\mu_B^2 + 4\mu_B\gamma\sigma_{H+B}^3 + \mu_B^4)\dots \end{array}\right]$$

Mathematical Appendix

Here, we derive Eq. (4.4b) in more detail. Define $V \equiv E[W(H_T)]$, the expected utility in period 1, conditional on survival to that period. The marginal rate of substitution can then be equivalently expressed as $\delta = \dfrac{V}{W'(\mu_H)}$, the ratio of marginal utility of increased LE to marginal utility of HRQoL in period 1.

We begin by proving the equivalence of two different formulations of TVMI:

$$\text{TVMI} = K\omega_H R\{\mu_p \phi \delta + \phi p_1 \mu_B \varepsilon\} \tag{A4.1}$$

$$\text{TVMI} = K\phi[\mu_p \rho H_0 + p_1 \omega_H R\mu_B \varepsilon] \tag{A4.2}$$

By inspection, we can see that this equivalence rests on the proposition that $\omega_H R\delta = \rho H_0$. To prove the latter, note that $\delta \equiv \left[\dfrac{E[W(H_T + B)]}{W'(\mu_H)}\right]$, $R \equiv \left[\dfrac{W'(\mu_H)}{W'(H_0)}\right]$, and $\omega_H \equiv \left[\dfrac{W'(H_0)H_0}{W(H_0)}\right]$. Therefore,

$$\omega_H R\delta = \left[\dfrac{W'(H_0)H_0}{W(H_0)}\right]\left[\dfrac{W'(\mu_H)}{W'(H_0)}\right]\left[\dfrac{E[W(H_T + B)]}{W'(\mu_H)}\right] = \dfrac{E[W(H_T + B)]}{W(H_0)}H_0.$$

Since $\rho \equiv \dfrac{E[W(H_T + B)]}{W(H_0)}$, the result follows, and Eqs. (A4.1) and (A4.2) are equivalent.

To estimate ρ, consider the Taylor series expansion of V around H_0:

$$E(V) \approx W(H_0) + W'(H_0)E(H_T - H_0)$$

$$+ \frac{1}{2}W''(H_0)E(H_T - H_0)^2 + \frac{1}{6}W'''(H_0)E(H_T - H_0)^3 + \dots \tag{A4.3}$$

Divide Eq. (A4.3) by $W(H_0)$, following the definition of ρ, and analyze it term by term:

$$\text{First Term}: \frac{W(H_0)}{W(H_0)} = 1 \qquad (A4.4)$$

The second term is $\dfrac{W'(H_0)E(H_T - H_0)}{W(H_0)}$. Multiply and divide this term by H_0, recognizing that the component parts are ω_H (defined at H_0) and $t^* \equiv \dfrac{H_0 - E(H_T)}{H_0}$, the expected relative loss in health status after treatment. With these definitions:

$$\text{Second Term}: -\omega_H t^* \qquad (A4.5)$$

The third term is $\dfrac{1}{2}\dfrac{W''(H_0)E(H_T - H_0)^2}{W(H_0)}$. Multiply and divide by $W'(H_0)H_0^2$, allocating one H_0 term to the numerator to convert absolute risk aversion, r, into relative risk aversion, r_H^*, and the other to complete ω_H. With these algebraic changes,

$$\text{Third Term}: -\frac{1}{2}\omega_H r_H^* t^{*2} \qquad (A4.6)$$

Note that r_H^* is measured at H_0.

The fourth term of Eq. (A4.3) is $\dfrac{1}{6}W'''(H_0)E(H_T - H_0)^3$. Dividing by $W(H_0)$ gives $\dfrac{1}{6}[W'''(H_0)E(H_T - H_0)^3]\dfrac{1}{W(H_0)}$. Multiply and divide by $W'(H_0)W''(H_0)H_0^3$. Then,

$$\text{Fourth Term}: -\frac{1}{6}\pi_H^* r_H^* \omega_H t^{*3} \qquad (A4.7)$$

As before, π_H^* is defined at H_0. Any fifth term involving kurtosis would follow the same general strategy.

In summation, the Taylor Series approximation to $\dfrac{V}{W(H_o)} \equiv \rho$ is

$$\rho \approx 1 - \omega_H \left[t^* + \frac{1}{2} r_H^* t^{*2} + \frac{1}{6} \pi_H^* r_H^* t^{*3} + \ldots \right] \qquad \text{(A4.8)}$$

Further Discussion of ψ

For the mathematically addicted, we add the following insight [while assuming that $W(0) = 0$]:

$$\psi = \frac{\dfrac{(W(H_0) - W(H_{0d}))}{(H_0 - H_{0d})}}{\dfrac{W(H_0) - W(0)}{H_0 - 0}}$$

This equation expresses ψ as the ratio of two slopes: (1) The average slope of W between $H_{0d} > 0$ and H_0; and (2) the average slope of W between 0 and H_0. For a strictly concave, increasing utility function, the slope between H_{0d} and H_0 will be strictly less than the slope between 0 and H_0. For a linear utility function, on the other hand, the slopes will be equal. This provides another way of demonstrating that ψ always declines as risk aversion increases, because greater risk aversion implies greater concavity in W. Furthermore, since $\psi \leq 1$ and $0 \leq d^* < 1$, the denominator of Eq. (5.4) is always positive, and therefore K_{GRACE} is always positive and well defined.

The Relationships Between Disability and Value of Improving
Quality of Life and Extending Life Expectancy

This appendix assesses mathematically the situations in which disability increases the value of extending LE. In standard CEA, increased disability *always* lowers the value of increased LE. In GRACE, just the opposite is true in many situations, which we explore next.

IMPROVEMENTS IN HRQOL

First, we show that permanent disability increases the WTP for improvements in average HRQoL. Eq. (5.4), combined with the measure of TVMI in Eq. (4.1a), implies that the marginal value of an improvement in average HRQoL is given by

$$\frac{K\omega_H R}{(1-\psi d^*)}\phi p_1 \varepsilon \tag{A5.1}$$

Greater disability increases $\dfrac{1}{1-\psi d^*}$, since d^* ranges from 0 (worst health) to 1 (perfect health) and the range of ψ is similarly limited. Moreover, if utility exhibits CRRA over HRQoL, all other terms are unaffected by disability. This provides an important benchmark for understanding these issues because utility in health is plausibly CRRA or nearly so. (The economics literature suggests that utility in consumption, C, is CRRA or nearly so.)

Technically, disability could have complex effects on ω_H, ψ, and ε, if relative risk aversion varies with HRQoL. In this case, the relationship between disability and HRQoL needs to be judged empirically. However, we know with certainty that R increases more than linearly with disability, and this may prove to be the dominant factor in assessing the full effects of disability on the value of improving average HRQoL.

EXTENDING LE

Turning to life extension, Eq. (4.1a) implies that the value of life extension, μ_p, is given by $K\omega_H R\mu_p\delta$. The total disability-adjusted value of life extension is thus given by

$$\text{TDVLE} \equiv \frac{K\omega_H R\mu_p\delta}{(1-\psi d^*)} \tag{A5.2}$$

Appendix 4.1 proved that $\delta = \dfrac{\rho H_0}{\omega_H R}$. Using the definition of ρ, this becomes $\delta = \dfrac{E(W(H_T))H_0}{W(H_0)\omega_H R}$. Moreover, by definition, $\dfrac{W(H_{0d})}{W(H_0)} = 1 - \psi d^*$. Substituting these two terms into TDVLE yields

$$\text{TDVLE} \equiv K\mu_p \frac{V}{W(H_{0d})} \tag{A5.3}$$

Exploiting the definition of $V \equiv E[W(H_{1S} + B)]$ from Chapter 4, this becomes

$$\text{TDVLE} \equiv K\mu_p \left[\frac{E[W(H_{1S} + B)]}{W(H_{0d})} \right] H_0 \tag{A5.4}$$

If permanent disability weakly increases $\dfrac{E(W(H_{1S} + B))}{W(H_{0d})}$, then TDVLE weakly rises (holding μ_p fixed), and vice versa.

Next, we show for illustrative purposes that people with disabilities have equal WTP for LE under CRRA utility and multiplicative disability as would otherwise-similar nondisabled people. To focus on the disability effects, assume that illness and treatment effects are nonstochastic. Assume further that utility belongs to the hyperbolic absolute risk aversion family. We implement multiplicative disability by assuming that $H_{0d} = H_0(1-d^*)$ and further that $H_{1S} + B = H_0(1-\ell_t^*)(1-d^*)$, where $0 < \ell_t^* < 1$ represents the percentage loss in HRQoL from acute treated illness and d^* continues to represent the percentage loss in HRQoL from disability. Define $\omega_H(H_{0d}) \equiv \dfrac{W'(H_{0d})H_{0d}}{W(H_{0d})}$ and $\omega_H(H_{1S} + B) \equiv \dfrac{W'(H_{1S} + B)(H_{1S} + B)}{W(H_{1S} + B)}$, the elasticities of utility with respect to HRQoL evaluated as indicated. Differentiation implies that

$$\frac{\partial}{\partial d^*}\left[\frac{W(H_{1S} + B)}{W(H_{0d})}\right]$$
$$= \frac{\left[W'(H_{0d})H_0 W(H_{1S} + B) - W'(H_{1S} + B)H_0(1-\ell_t^*)W(H_{0d})\right]}{W(H_{0d})^2}$$

$$(A.5.5a)$$

This can be simplified as

$$\frac{\partial}{\partial d^*}\left[\frac{W(H_{1S} + B)}{W(H_{0d})}\right]$$
$$= W(H_{0d})W(H_{1S} + B)$$
$$\times \frac{\left[\dfrac{W'(H_{0d})H_{0d}}{W(H_{0d})}\dfrac{H_0}{H_{0d}} - \dfrac{W'(H_{1S} + B)(H_{1S} + B)}{W(H_{1S} + B)}\dfrac{H_0(1-\ell_t^*)}{H_{1S} + B}\right]}{W(H_{0d})^2} \quad (A5.5b)$$

Now, observe that by definition, $\dfrac{H_0}{H_{0d}} = \dfrac{1}{1-d^*} = \dfrac{H_0(1-t^*)}{H_{1S} + B}$. Furthermore, when utility is CRRA, the elasticity of utility is also constant so that $\dfrac{W'(H_{0d})H_{0d}}{W(H_{0d})} = \dfrac{W'(H_{1S} + B)(H_{1S} + B)}{W(H_{1S} + B)}$. It thus follows that

$\frac{\partial}{\partial d^*}\left[\frac{W(H_{1S}+B)}{W(H_{0d})}\right]=0$. This proves the result that TDVLE does not vary with d^* as long as utility exhibits CRRA in H and disability is modeled multiplicatively.

Finally, we derive sufficient conditions under which permanent disability increases $\dfrac{E(W(H_{1S}+B))}{W(H_{0d})}$, and hence TDVLE. This is the condition

to prove that the value of extending a person's life expectancy is greater than it would be for an otherwise-similar nondisabled person. Consider the Taylor series expansion of $E(W(H_{1S}+B))$ around H_{0d}. Following the same approach used in Appendix I.A and Appendix I.B in Lakdawalla and Phelps (2022), one can show that

$$
\frac{E(W(H_{1S}+B))}{W(H_{0d})}=1-\omega_H\left(\frac{t^*-d^*}{1-d^*}\right)-\omega_H r_H^*\left(\frac{t^*-d^*}{1-d^*}\right)^2-\omega_H r_H^* \pi_H^*\left(\frac{t^*-d^*}{1-d^*}\right)^3-\ldots
$$

$$
=1-\omega_H\left(\frac{t^*-d^*}{1-d^*}\right)\left[1+r_H^*\left(\frac{t^*-d^*}{1-d^*}\right)+r_H^*\pi_H^*\left(\frac{t^*-d^*}{1-d^*}\right)^2-\ldots\right] \qquad \text{(A5.6)}
$$

Note that in this case, the relative risk preference terms are evaluated at H_{0d}. Under CRRA preferences, the relative risk preference terms do not vary with d^*. In this case, it is clear that $\dfrac{\partial}{\partial d^*}\dfrac{E(W(H_{1S}+B))}{W(H_{0d})}\geq 0$ if and only if $\dfrac{\partial}{\partial d^*}\left(\dfrac{t^*-d^*}{1-d^*}\right)\leq 0$. So, when does this situation occur?

$$
\frac{\partial}{\partial d^*}\left(\frac{t^*-d^*}{1-d^*}\right)=\frac{\left(\dfrac{\partial t^*}{\partial d^*}-1\right)(1-d^*)+(t^*-d^*)}{(1-d^*)^2} \qquad \text{(A5.7a)}
$$

This derivative will be weakly negative (≤ 0) if and only if

$$
\frac{\partial t^*}{\partial d^*}\leq\frac{1-t^*}{1-d^*}\leq 1 \qquad \text{(A5.7b)}
$$

Equation (A5.7b) requires that increased disability lowers HRQoL in the sick state by less than in the healthy state. For curative therapies, we know for sure that $\dfrac{\partial t^*}{\partial d^*} \leq 1$ is always true, but for less than perfect therapies, the requirement becomes nontrivial.

A useful alternate formulation of this expression arises from the change of variables, $D \equiv 1 - d^*$ and $T \equiv 1 - t^*$. D and T represent the HRQoL index in the healthy and treated sick states, respectively, in the presence of disability. Notice that $\left(\dfrac{t^* - d^*}{1 - d^*}\right) = \left(\dfrac{D - T}{D}\right) = 1 - \dfrac{T}{D}$. Moreover, $\dfrac{\partial}{\partial D}\left(\dfrac{D - T}{D}\right) = -\dfrac{\left(\dfrac{\partial T}{\partial D}D - T\right)}{D^2}$. Observe that $\dfrac{\partial}{\partial D}\left(\dfrac{D - T}{D}\right) \leq 0$ if and only if $\left(\dfrac{\partial T}{\partial D}\dfrac{D}{T}\right) \geq 1$. In other words, reducing disability so that healthy state HRQoL rises by 1 percent must increase treated sick state QoL by more than 1 percent in order to have the situation in which greater disability increases WTP for extensions in HRQoL.

This condition interacts with the way analysts combine disability and acute illness. In the multiplicative approach, final health is measured as $(1 - d^*)(1 - \ell^*)$. This ensures that increased disability lowers HRQoL in the sick state by less than in the healthy state. In the additive approach, where final health is measured as $(1 - d^* - \ell^*)$, this cannot be ensured. This also involves any potential interaction between disability and the treatment that improves the acute illness, thereby shifting the effect of the illness from ℓ^* to t^*.

Note: This appendix extensively uses the mathematical derivations in Appendix I.C of Lakdawalla and Phelps (2022).

Exact Estimation of GRACE

In some cases, analysts may have access to estimates of the underlying utility function for health-related quality of life, $W(H)$. This enables exact estimates of GRACE results, without need of Taylor series approximations. Here, we present the formulae for exact estimation, and we show how they relate to the GRACE approximation formulae that we have presented elsewhere in this book.

In what follows, we will use formulas such as $EW(H_{sj} + B_j)$ to represent the expected utility of the treatment in period j. This assumes that an exact equation has been chosen to represent $W(H)$. For example, if the CRRA formula is chosen, then $W(H) = \dfrac{H^\gamma}{\gamma}$. Of course, more complex versions of $W(H)$ can also be used if the parameters are known. For example, if the expo-power (EP) function is chosen, then $W(H) = 1 - e^{-(\gamma H^C)} = \dfrac{e^{(\gamma H^C)} - 1}{e^{(\gamma H^C)}}$, where both γ and C have been estimated using proper methods and data. The approach is the same, no matter what the chosen function for $W(H)$.

Computing expected utilities is straightforward at this point. Using randomized controlled trial data as an example, each participant's health status can be determined using standard methods such as EQ-5 or PROMIS, mapping them directly to a single scale of health, comparable to a visual analog scale (VAS) health measure. The utility function then converts these health measures to utilities. Then, expected utility tells us that value is linear in utility, so we only need to compute the average of such utilities to determine values such as ρ requires.

We also note that using discrete choice experiment (DCE) data to estimate risk parameters requires that analysts assume a specific utility function to calculate certainty equivalents (CEs). This means that the same analysis used to estimate risk parameters can identify the best-fit utility function among those tested. Thus, when risk preference data are acquired using DCE methods, the exact method for calculating GRACE values will likely be the most useful. See Appendix 8.1 for details of this approach.

ESTIMATION OF INCREMENTAL COSTS

To fix ideas, we remind the reader how to estimate incremental costs in a multi-period setting. Define Cost_j^T as the cost incurred by the treated group in period j, and define Cost_j^U as the cost incurred by the untreated (i.e., comparator) group in period j. Define the one-period discount factor as β. Define p_j^T as the probability of surviving from period 0 to period j in the treated group, and define p_j^U as the probability of surviving from period 0 to period j in the untreated group. Define ϕ as the probability of falling ill in period one.

The incremental period 0 expected net present cost of the treatment is given by

$$\text{Cost}_0 \equiv \phi \sum_{j=0}^{\infty} \beta^j \{ p_j^T \text{Cost}_j^T - p_n^U \text{Cost}_j^U \}$$

Defining $\Delta \text{Cost}_j \equiv \text{Cost}_j^T - \text{Cost}_j^U$ and $\mu_{pj} \equiv p_j^T - p_j^U$, this is equivalent to

$$\text{Cost}_0 = \phi \sum_{j=0}^{\infty} \beta^j \{ p_j^T \text{Cost}_j^T - p_j^U \text{Cost}_j^T + p_j^U \text{Cost}_j^T - p_j^U \text{Cost}_j^U \}$$

$$= \phi \sum_{j=0}^{\infty} \beta^j \{ \mu_{pj} \text{Cost}_j^T + p_j^U \Delta \text{Cost}_j \}$$

EXACT ESTIMATION OF INCREMENTAL BENEFITS

Now turn to the benefits of the technology. Recall that period 0 health loss due to permanent disability satisfies $0 \leq d^* < 1$, and period 0 health is $H_0(1 - d^*)$. Define H_{sj} as stochastic period j health in the untreated sick state; recall that these health levels are inclusive of any preexisting permanent disability. Define the stochastic period j health improvement as B_j; this also incorporates any effects of preexisting permanent disability.

In keeping with the conventional cost-effectiveness approach, we assume that people are perfectly insured against health shocks and perfectly annuitized. Therefore, consumption in period j is given by $c_j = c$, which is independent of the illness and treatment state. Implicit in this assumption is another: The cost of the technology is assumed too small to affect period 0 consumption, which remains at c. In other words, the purchase of the new technology does not introduce income effects that influence the period 0 marginal utility of consumption.

If health in period j is given by H_j, define period j utility as $U(c)W(H_j)$. The period 0 expected incremental benefit of the technology is thus

$$\frac{\phi}{U'(c)W(H_0(1-d^*))} \sum_{j=0}^{\infty} \beta^j U(c)\{p_j^T EW(H_{sj} + B_j) - p_j^U EW(H_{sj})\}$$

Recalling that $K \equiv \dfrac{U(c)}{U'(c)H_0}$, we can write this expression equivalently as

$$\frac{\phi K H_0}{W(H_0(1-d^*))} \sum_{j=0}^{\infty} \beta^j \{p_j^T EW(H_{sj} + B_j) - p_j^U EW(H_{sj})\}$$

Some additional algebraic manipulation reveals

$$\frac{\phi K H_0}{W(H_0(1-d^*))} \sum_{j=0}^{\infty} \beta^j \left\{ \begin{array}{l} p_j^T EW(H_{sj} + B_j) - p_j^U EW(H_{sj} + B_j) \\ + p_j^U EW(H_{sj} + B_j) - p_j^U EW(H_{sj}) \end{array} \right\}$$

$$= \frac{\phi K H_0}{W(H_0(1-d^*))} \sum_{j=0}^{\infty} \beta^j \left\{ \begin{array}{l} \mu_{pj}[EW(H_{sj} + B_j)] \\ + p_j^U [EW(H_{sj} + B_j) - EW(H_{sj})] \end{array} \right\}$$

EXACT ESTIMATION OF NET MONETARY BENEFITS

Combining the results above allows us to compute the exact net monetary benefit of the technology in question:

$$
\text{TVMI}^{\text{Exact}} = \phi \sum_{j=0}^{\infty} \beta^j \left\{ K \left[\begin{array}{c} \mu_{pj} \dfrac{[EW(H_{sj} + B_j)]}{W(H_0(1-d^*))} H_0 \\[2ex] + p_j^U \dfrac{[EW(H_{sj} + B_j) - EW(H_{sj})]}{W(H_0(1-d^*))} H_0 \\[2ex] -[\mu_{pj}\text{Cost}_j^T + p_j^U \Delta\text{Cost}_j] \end{array} \right] \right\}
$$

EXACT ESTIMATION OF INCREMENTAL GENERALIZED COST-EFFECTIVENESS RATIO

Recall that $K \equiv \dfrac{U(c)}{U'(c)H_0}$, $\omega_H \equiv \dfrac{W'(H_0)}{W(H_0)} H_0$, $R_j \equiv \dfrac{W'(E(H_{sj}))}{W'(H_0)}$, and $(1-d^*\psi) \equiv \dfrac{W(H_0(1-d^*))}{W(H_0)}$. Recalling further that $\mu_{Hj} \equiv E(H_{sj})$, it follows that $\dfrac{K\omega_H R_j}{1-d^*\psi} = \dfrac{U(c)W'(\mu_{Hj})}{U'(c)W(H_0(1-d^*))}$, which represents the period 0 WTP for a unit change in average period j HRQoL. Notice that all the parameters within this WTP term are known exactly by the analyst in the case in which the function W is known. For any reference time period i, we can rewrite $\text{TVMI}^{\text{Exact}}$ as

$$
\text{TVMI}^{\text{Exact}} = \phi \sum_{j=0}^{\infty} \beta^j \left\{ \dfrac{K\omega_H R_i}{1-d^*\psi} \dfrac{1-d^*\psi}{K\omega_H R_i} \left[\begin{array}{c} \mu_{pj} \dfrac{[EW(H_{sj} + B_j)]}{W(H_0(1-d^*))} H_0 \\[2ex] + p_j^U \dfrac{[EW(H_{sj} + B_j) - EW(H_{sj})]}{W(H_0(1-d^*))} H_0 \end{array} \right] \right.
$$
$$
\left. -[\mu_{pj}\text{Cost}_j^T + p_j^U \Delta\text{Cost}_j] \right\}
$$

Therefore, TVMI > 0 if and only if

$$\frac{K\omega_H R_i}{1-d^*\psi} > \frac{\sum_{j=0}^{\infty}\beta^j[\mu_{pj}\text{Cost}_j^T + p_j^U\Delta\text{Cost}_j]}{\sum_{j=0}^{\infty}\beta^j\left\{\frac{1-d^*\psi}{K\omega_H R_i}\left[\mu_{pj}\frac{[EW(H_{sj}+B_j)]}{W(H_0(1-d^*))}H_0 + p_j^U\frac{[EW(H_{sj}+B_j)-EW(H_{sj})]}{W(H_0(1-d^*))}H_0\right]\right\}}$$

The left-hand side represents the incremental generalized risk-adjusted cost-effectiveness ratio, in its exact form.

RELATIONSHIP BETWEEN EXACT AND APPROXIMATED ESTIMATES

We now discuss the relationship between the "exact" form and GRACE's derived approximations. For notational simplicity, we conduct this analysis for a single period, j. We also focus on the net monetary benefit formulation because the IGRACER formulation is shown above to be equivalent to the net monetary benefit formulation.

Longevity Extensions

The discounted period j value of longevity extension is given above by

$$\phi K\mu_{pj}\beta^j\frac{[EW(H_{sj}+B_j)]}{W(H_0(1-d^*))}H_0$$

Recall $\rho_j \equiv \frac{[E[W(H_{Sj}+B_j)]]}{W(H_0)}$. Therefore, the value of longevity extension in period j is equivalent to

$$\phi K\mu_{pj}\rho_j H_0$$

When the function $W(H)$ is unknown, ρ_j can be approximated via Taylor series methods.

Quality of Life Improvements

Above, we showed that the discounted value of a period j HRQoL improvement is given by

$$EV(B_j) \equiv \beta^j \frac{U(C)(p_j^U \phi E[W(H_{sj} + B_j) - W(H_{sj})])}{U'(C)W(H_0(1 - d^*))}$$

Using the definition of K, we can rewrite this as

$$EV(B_j) \equiv \beta^j K \phi p_j^U \frac{(E[W(H_{sj} + B_j) - W(H_{sj})])}{W(H_0(1 - d^*))} H_0$$

Based on the definitions of ω_H, R_p and $(1 - d^* \psi)$, $\dfrac{\omega_H R}{1 - d^* \psi} = \dfrac{W'(\mu_{Hj})}{W(H_0(1 - d^*))} H_0$. As a result, we can rewrite $EV(B_j)$ as

$$EV(B_j) \equiv \beta^j K \phi p_j^U \frac{\omega_H R}{1 - d^* \psi} \frac{(E[W(H_{sj} + B_j) - W(H_{sj})])}{W'(\mu_{Hj})}$$

Notice that $\dfrac{(E[W(H_{sj} + B_j) - W(H_{sj})])}{W'(\mu_{Hj})}$ represents the gain in average HRQoL due to the technology; in other words, this ratio is the marginal rate of substitution between the technology and HRQoL. Elsewhere, we have defined this concept as the incremental generalized risk-adjusted QALY, which is approximated by $\mu_{Bj} \varepsilon_j \approx \dfrac{(E[W(H_{sj} + B_j) - W(H_{sj})])}{W'(\mu_{Hj})}$. This illustrates that the exact estimation formula can be approximated by

$$EV(B_j) \equiv K \phi p_j^U \frac{\omega_H R}{1 - d^* \psi} \mu_B \varepsilon$$

Estimation of Discrete Choice Experiment Parameters
Using Maximum Likelihood Estimation

Regarding estimation of these DCE models, we note that there are two ways to carry out MLE analysis. In one approach (random utility models), the error term is attached to the utility level. In the other, the error term is attached to the parameter value (random preference models). Apesteguia and Ballester (2014, 2018) specifically discuss that the random utility model has embedded biases that distort inferences about relative risk aversion. Specifically, individuals with higher levels of risk aversion may choose riskier gambles with higher probability, thus biasing downward the estimated risk version level. Using random preference models avoids this bias. They provide specific mathematical models to properly estimate random preference models that can serve as a guide to researchers pursuing such studies in the realm of risk aversion in H. They specifically discusses such estimation in a multiparameter model such as would arise if using EP or HARA utility models.

Preface

1. https://cevr.tuftsmedicalcenter.org/databases/cea-registry.
2. https://www.cms.gov/About-CMS/Agency-Information/OMH/resource-center/hcps-and-researchers/Improving-Access-to-Care-for-People-with-Disabilities.
3. The following discussion presumes that diminishing returns to health prevail, so that people are risk averse. As we discuss later, severely ill patients may actually be risk-seeking, not risk-averse.

Chapter 1

1. Rusted out heap of the month.
2. In economic jargon, we would need to ascertain the equivalent variation—the amount of money that would make a person just as happy (on the same indifference curve) as if the illness had not occurred.
3. Other issues enter individual decisions about such tests, including (among others) familial history, individuals' fear of cancer, beliefs about the value of testing, etc.
4. Pronounced "kwa-lees." In principle, GRACE is agnostic about the measure of health used. Other health-measurement approaches are admissible within GRACE.
5. https://professional.heart.org/en/science-news/acc-aha-statement-on-cost-value-methodology-in-clinical-practice-guidelines-and-performance-measures/ Commentary, last visited September 1, 2023.
6. Chapter 7 reviews extensively different methods to estimate the proper threshold.
7. For a more extensive discussion of this practice, see Chapter 14 in Phelps and Parente (2017).
8. https://www.ajmc.com/view/availability-of-prices-for-shoppable-services-on-hospital-internet-sites, last visited September 1, 2023.
9. Many U.S. hospitals inserted special computer code into their websites that limited access to these data, thus preventing other organizations from "harvesting" the data and summarizing them in various ways. In July 2021, the Biden administration proposed to increase the penalty for noncompliance up to $2 million per year.

10. In other areas of economics, externalities include pollution, traffic congestion, groundwater pumping rates, and even the extent of comparison shopping undertaken by individuals.

11. In our development of GRACE, all of the probability measures are "known" with certainty. We did this deliberately to reduce complexity of the model. But one could readily make these probability estimates uncertain, in which case the GRACE model would directly provide measures of the value, for example, of improved diagnostic certainty. In some sense, the best way to think about this in the current GRACE framework is to think of "uncertainty of treatment outcome" as the combined effects of incomplete or incorrect diagnosis, coupled with intrinsic uncertainty in the outcomes of the treatment, given a correct diagnosis.

CHAPTER 2

1. The wording on some of these "standard gamble" methods is potentially disturbing. Some ask respondents to anchor their utility evaluations on two states of the world: (1) perfect health and (2) "instant and painless death." Setting aside how different religious beliefs might affect views of the second alternative, we believe that no research subject has ever experienced at least the second, if not both, of these health states, making a utility evaluation using this wording somewhat problematic.

2. We review the more-extensive PROMIS system developed by the U.S. National Institutes of Health in more detail in Chapter 9.

3. The term "utility" is a bit odd in modern language use because it implies "usefulness" or "functionality." As it was originally developed by Jeremy Bentham, John Stuart Mill, and others, it meant "happiness" in the context of their "utilitarian" philosophy of economic thinking. We intend to equate "utility" to "happiness" throughout.

4. Chapter 8 explores "happiness economic" methods to help understand the role of health in creating happiness. This approach uses people's own stated values of their level of happiness as a key input.

5. Later, we will break apart H into two components, HRQoL and LE. That set of trade-offs has its own important and interesting issues to consider.

6. For those uninitiated to "Yogi-isms," see https://en.wikipedia.org/wiki/Yogi_Be rra#%22Yogi-isms%22 (last visited August 1, 2022).

7. This is the precise measure derived in Phelps (2019), discussed in more detail in Chapter 7 in this volume.

8. Note that standard CEA is a special case of GRACE. If one assumes that $\omega_C = 1$, then that also implies that $R = 1$, in which case K_{GRACE} and K are identical.

9. The concept of risk aversion was discovered independently by Kenneth J Arrow and John W. Pratt. Pratt published his discovery first, in 1964, "Risk Aversion in the Small and in the Large"; Arrow's discovery was subsequently published in notes of a series of lectures he had given in 1965 in Helsinki as Chapter 2 of *Essays in the Theory of Risk-Bearing* (1971). Although Pratt was clearly the first to "publish," his 1964 article acknowledges his awareness of Arrow's previous discovery of the risk aversion concept.

10. Kimball's (1990) title, "Precautionary Savings in the Small and in the Large," clearly refers to Pratt's (1964) earlier title, "Risk Aversion in the Small and in the Large." Pratt grappled with risk aversion "in the large" because he did not have the tools to discuss how risk aversion changes as income changes. Using Kimball's 1990 work, Phelps (2022b) shows that if one can measure the higher order risk preference terms, then it becomes straightforward to understand how relative risk aversion behaves "in the large."

11. Brook Taylor, an Englishman, published *Incremental Methods, Direct and Indirect* in 1715. The original was, of course, written and titled in Latin. A highly regarded mathematician, he was part of a committee of England's Royal Society helping resolve disputes between Sir Isaac Newton and German mathematician Gottfried Wilhelm Leibnitz about their parallel discoveries in creating the calculus, one of the most fundamentally important inventions in human history.

12. Appendix 2.2 discusses convergence properties of the Taylor series expansion in Eq. (2.9).

13. Indeed, integral calculus formulas calculate this area based on the asymptotic limit as the width of each rectangle goes to zero.

14. Appendix 2.2 discusses convergence properties of this integral.

15. Comparing results from the Taylor series method (for details, see Table 11.1) and the numerical integration method (see Table 2.2) reveals the extent of possible overestimation from the numerical integration approach. The most extreme value in Table 2.2 appears at the lower right-hand corner ($r_H^* = 1$ and $\ell^* = 0.9$). The numerical integration value from Table 2.2 is 2.39, whereas the fully converged Taylor series value in Table 11.1 is 2.28. Therefore, the greatest relative error in Table 2.2 is 4.8 percent, and most of the values in Table 2.2 are equivalent to at least two decimal places to comparable values using Eq. (2.11c).

CHAPTER 3

1. Recall that r_C^* is the income elasticity of the marginal utility of income. Much of the literature on risk discusses whether r_C^* has constant relative risk aversion (CRRA), increasing relative risk aversion (IRRA), or decreasing relative risk aversion (DRRA). This means, of course, that we are interested in how fast an elasticity (r_C^*) changes as C changes, so we are discussing the income elasticity of an income elasticity. Although this may seem weird at first, it turns out that the CRRA/IRRA/DRRA issue is quite important when looking at r_H^*, as we explore in detail in Chapter 9.

2. Throughout this discussion, to simplify exposition at little loss of generality, we assume hyperbolic absolute risk aversion (HARA) utility, as discussed in Chapter 8 in detail.

3. See Appendix 3.1 for expanded analysis of this term.

4. The $\frac{1}{2}$ comes from the standard Taylor series expansion (i.e., $\frac{1}{2!}$).

5. As before, the $\frac{1}{6}$ term comes from the Taylor series expansion (it is 1/3!).

6. If r_H^* is constant for all values of H, then $\pi^* = 1 + r_H^*$, so, for example, if $r_H^* = 1, \pi^* = 2$.

7. Once more, the $\frac{1}{24}$ term comes from the Taylor series expansion because $24 = 4!$

8. To be clear, we are not asserting that real-world treatments will necessarily have outcomes well-described by the β distribution. Rather, we use the β distribution because it conveniently captures the essential features of GRACE that we need.

9. Doubling both β and α reduces skewness by approximately 25 percent.

10. In both of these equations, the risk parameters are measured at untreated health levels.

CHAPTER 4

1. https://www.nhlbi.nih.gov/health/educational/lose_wt/BMI/bmicalc.htm, Last visited September 1, 2023.

CHAPTER 5

1. We assume throughout that $H_{1W} = H_{0d}$ so that permanent disability persists from period 0 onwards. This generalization also requires that H_{1S} include permanent disability; therefore, analysts must calculate H_{1s} to reflect the effects of untreated acute illness and any preexisting permanent disability.

2. See Appendix 5.1 for an additional discussion of ψ.

3. This is a literature with which we have little familiarity. Searching the terms "assimilative coping" and "adaptive coping" will guide the interested reader toward it.

CHAPTER 6

1. Although we suppress the extra notation, note that variance and skewness in both the treatment and comparator arms should also be estimated in each period, in addition to the differences in variance and skewness across arms. In addition, we presume that permanent disability is fixed over time and that any variation in it could be represented using additional time-series variation in $d_n^*, \ell_n^*,$ and $t_n^*.$

CHAPTER 7

1. The per capita GDP in 1991 was \$19,900 (https://fred.stlouisfed.org/series/PCAGD PGBA646NWDB), and the exchange rate averaged approximately 1.8:1 during 1991 (https://www.poundsterlinglive.com/bank-of-england-spot/historical-spot-exchange-rates/gbp/GBP-to-USD-1991). Therefore, per capita GDP in the United Kingdom was approximately £11,000.

2. https://www.epa.gov/environmental-economics/mortality-risk-valuation, last visited June 5, 2021.

3. For a simple exposition of the problem, see https://en.wikipedia.org/wiki/Omit ted-variable_bias.

4. Boundedness may actually be the only sensible way to think about utility of consumption. If utility for any commodity or good (e.g., blueberries) is unbounded,

then there exists some finite quantity of blueberries that the individual would happily accept in exchange for most, and perhaps all, other food, or even all other goods and services.

5. As Phelps and Cinatl (2021) show, if the $\dfrac{K}{C}$ ratio rises faster than 1:1 with income, this implies that utility of consumption has declining relative risk aversion (DRRA).

6. https://www.cms.gov/Research-Statistics-Data-and-Systems/Statistics-Trends-and-Reports/NationalHealthExpendData/NationalHealthAccountsHistorical.

CHAPTER 8

1. Readers who are not involved in estimation of these utility parameters may wish to skip or just skim this chapter, but even for those readers, we hope that this chapter will assist in understanding how the key GRACE parameters can be estimated.

2. To appreciate this relationship, consider a single-good utility function, $U(C)$. Here, by definition, $\omega_C \equiv \dfrac{U'(C)C}{U(C)}$. If U is strictly concave and monotonic, it will be true that $U'(C)C < U(C)$ and thus that $\omega_C < 1$. For a simple example of this rule, note that when $U(C) = C^{1-\gamma}$, $U'(C) = (1-\gamma)C^{-\gamma}$, so $CU'(C) = (1-\gamma)C^{1-\gamma} = (1-\gamma)U(C)$. Since positive but diminishing marginal utility requires that $0 < \gamma < 1$, $CU'(C) < U(C)$.

3. When $b < 0$, this formulation closely resembles the widely used Stone–Geary utility function, wherein b is taken to be a minimum "required level" of consumption, and below which level, utility is either undefined or equals 0.

4. Another way to do this without assuming that $a = 1$ is to scale b by a so that $\dfrac{b}{a} = b^*$. Then, $r_H^*(H) = (1-\gamma)\left[\dfrac{H}{H+b^*}\right]$.

5. If discussing the utility of consumption, which can in concept grow without limits, $r_H^* + \omega_H$ asymptotically approaches 1 as C grows very large, and as this occurs, r_C^* asymptotically approaches $(1-\gamma)$ and ω_C asymptotically approaches γ.

6. See Appendix 2.2, which discusses issues about Taylor series convergence.

7. https://www.gallup.com/analytics/318875/global-research.aspx. The current editors are at the University of British Columbia, Columbia University, Oxford University, and the London School of Economics.

8. Some people frame the happiness question to respondents as a series of intervals, from which they choose one option (e.g., $0 \le$ happy < 1, $1 \le$ happy < 2, . . ., $9 \le$ happy $= 10$). This "discrete choice" framework alters the econometric estimation techniques required, but not the basic concept. For this discussion, we presume that a continuous measure of happiness has been reported by the respondents.

9. Recall that our basic model states that the utilities of health and consumption are "separable," but even in this environment, the marginal utility of consumption depends on the level of health and conversely.

10. The standard error of the key ratio will be determined by the standard error of the difference between β_1 and β_3 if the second-order terms do not differ from 0. A similar but more complicated estimate arises if β_2 and/or β_4 differ from 0.

11. This is the principal utility function used by Holt and Laury (2002), which we discuss later.

12. They conducted one experiment with higher stakes to test whether the magnitude of money involved affected the risk aversion level. In that experiment, $x = 135$, $y = 90$, and $z = 30$.

13. A possible exception is in the analysis of pain using the cold pressor test (Schosser et al., 2016). These tests involve immersing the subjects' hand in very cold water to experimentally inflict pain, which can vary over both duration and degree (colder water temperature) of pain.

CHAPTER 9

1. By contrast, the health utilities index specifically uses standard gamble methods to convert health status into utilities in the second phase of constructing their health index. That second step would make it inappropriate for use in GRACE. For details, see https://hqlo.biomedcentral.com/articles/10.1186/1477-7525-1-54.

2. For a brief presentation of this method, see https://www.publichealth.columbia.edu/research/population-health-methods/item-response-theory; last visited November 28, 2021.

3. If the attributes are measured on different scales, a mechanism to convert them to a common scale is necessary. For a discussion of this issue within MAUT, see Keeney (1974) and Edwards and Barron (1994). This would not be an issue with PROMIS because it uses a 1–5 scale for each item. The MAUT structure developed in Keeney (1974) relies wholly on linear transformations.

4. https://cevr.tuftsmedicalcenter.org/databases/cea-registry.

5. Again, we remind the reader about the possibility of using exact utility functions, as elaborated in Chapter 2 relating to the estimation of the severity adjustment R.

6. In this instance, higher order risk parameters should be estimated using HARA utility as discussed in Chapter 8.

7. Recall from Chapter 5 that this ratio of utilities is the proper adjustment because the marginal utility of consumption in the baseline (pre-illness) period, which crucially measures the "opportunity cost" of improving health, equals $U'(C_0)W(H_0)$ without disability. The adjustment replaces $W(H_0)$ with the proper value $W(H_{0d})$, which incorporates disability.

8. This can be generalized to non-CRRA utility, but doing so complicates the exposition of the basic concepts with no gain in understanding of the effects of disability on WTP.

9. Suppose that the disease annual incidence and the permanent disability prevalence each occur with a probability of 1 per 1,000 people. Then the joint probability of their occurring in any year is $\left[\dfrac{1}{1,000}\right]^2$, the proverbial "one in a million" occurrence. In the United States, with approximately 240 million adults, the maximum potential set of respondents would be 240 people per year. For diseases or disabilities that are age-limited in incidence or prevalence (e.g., pediatric diseases), that number would fall accordingly.

10. If utility is not CRRA, assuming the more general HARA provides methods to allow the increment in the risk parameter to differ from 1.0, with the amount depending on whether utility is DRRA or IRRA.

11. If consumers are risk-preferring—for example, in very bleak health states—then *more* variance will be desirable.

12. In addition to the truncated Taylor series terms, we remind readers that Eq. (9.6) involves an approximation as discussed in the footnote regarding Eq. (3.1). This expansion of detail in the approximation matters most for large values of μ_B.

CHAPTER 10

1. A medical center leader known to one of us once whimsically stated that a "poorly understood medical fact was that there is a $1,000 bill in the colon of every adult American."

2. For example, if older people experience, on average, more severe illness, GRACE would prescribe higher values for treating the old than the young; thus, valuation may depend on how long a person has already lived, but in this example, GRACE produces the opposite conclusion from the "fair innings" approach.

3. https://icer.org.

4. The most generous of these "Medigap" plans almost entirely eliminates co-payments for enrolled customers but, of course, at the highest monthly premium for that coverage.

CHAPTER 11

1. Ramsey was a brilliant economist and mathematician who died in 1930 at age 26 years due to chronic liver disease, possibly as a result of undiagnosed leptospirosis, a bacterial infection that could easily have been cured by penicillin. Unfortunately, the curative properties of penicillin were only then being investigated in the laboratory of Scottish physician Alexander Fleming, but because it was so difficult to isolate and reproduce, he could not convince people that penicillin had any large-scale value. The first patient successfully treated with the drug consumed half of the known world supply at the time (1942). The first large-scale commercial production of penicillin was led by chemical engineer Margaret Hutchinson Rousseau (Madhavan, 2016). Although she became the first woman to be admitted into the American Institute of Chemical Engineers, she never received the sort of recognition that Fleming's earlier laboratory work received (a Nobel Prize in Medicine).

2. The assumption here is that higher prices today cause innovators to infer the likelihood of higher prices in the future, when they might bring their products to market. Consistent and clearly defined laws, policies, and administrative practices about drug pricing support this inference.

3. For simplicity, we abstract from treatments used in multiple indications with different severity levels. In practice, one can think of treatment j specifically as a treatment–indication pair.

4. The values in Table 11.1 are all exact to three decimal places (reported in two places). Comparison with Table 2.2 shows that the numerical integration method slightly overstates the integral values at the highest values of r_H^* and ℓ^*. At the extreme lower right corner ($r_H^* = 1$ and $\ell^* = 0.9$) the numerical approximation (= 2.39) overstates the Taylor series measure (= 2.28) by 4.8 percent.

5. For those deeply into the math, the different mixes of r_H^* and ω_H that add up to a total of 1.3 come about through changes in the HARA parameter γ, since $\omega_H = \left(\dfrac{\gamma}{1-\gamma}\right) r_H^*$ in HARA utility.

6. In brief, this model uses the product of medical spending on the intervention and the square of the coefficient of variation in its use. More variability signals uncertainty (or at least disagreement) about a technology's proper use.

7. The Institute of Medicine is now the National Academy of Medicine.

8. Here, we intend to include such things as surgical interventions and even different cognitive treatment strategies for patients that do not necessarily involve interventional therapeutics or biopharmaceutical products.

CHAPTER 12

1. The formal criterion states that a project's beneficiaries could, *in concept*, provide sufficient monetary compensation to "losers" from the project's implementation that they too were made better off, even though such compensation need not actually occur. Another way of stating this is that the net gain in consumer surplus across all members of society is positive.

2. Harsanyi, born in Hungary, emigrated to the United States after World War II and received a second PhD in economics under Kenneth Arrow at Stanford University. Harsanyi shared the Nobel Prize in Economics in 1994 (along with Richard Selten and John Nash) for his seminal work on game theory, but his contributions to welfare economics could be viewed as equally important. The two topics are related by the concept of uncertainty. His game-theoretic work focused on economic "games of incomplete information." His pathbreaking paper in 1955 on welfare economics focused on ways to describe economic welfare when uncertainty is present.

3. https://www.nice.org.uk/Media/Default/Get-involved/Meetings-In-Public/Public-board-meetings/nov-22-pbm-CHTE-methods-process-and-topic-selection.docx.

4. https://www.regjeringen.no/contentassets/d5da48ca5d1a4b128c72fc5daa3b4fd8/summary_the_magnussen_report_on_severity.pdf.

CHAPTER 13

1. Others in the health economics literature use constant absolute risk aversion (CARA) utility functions, which have been widely discarded in studies of financial risk (Phelps, 2022a). Assuming that similar issues exist in the analysis of utility in health, we recommend against using CARA utility to measure $W(H)$.

2. If sample sizes permit, adding estimates of the kurtosis in outcome distributions has added value, but the sample sizes to estimate kurtosis with adequate precision may lie beyond the sample size ranges for typical health technology evaluations.

3. https://www.fda.gov/drugs/new-drugs-fda-cders-new-molecular-entities-and-new-therapeutic-biological-products/new-drug-therapy-approvals-2020.

REFERENCES

Acemoglu D, Linn J. Market size in innovation: Theory and evidence from the pharmaceutical industry. *Quarterly Journal of Economics* 2004; 119(3): 1049–1090.

Adler MD. The puzzle of ex ante efficiency: Does rational approvability have moral weight? *University of Pennsylvania Law Review* 2002; 151: 1255–1290.

Al MJ, Feenstra TL, van Hout BA. Optimal allocation of resources over health care programmes: Dealing with decreasing marginal utility and uncertainty. *Health Economics* 2005; 14: 655–667.

Apesteguia J, Ballester MA. *Discrete choice estimation of risk aversion*. Barcelona Graduate School of Economics; September 2014.

Apesteguia J, Ballester MA. Monotone stochastic choice models: The case of risk and time preference. *Journal of Political Economy* 2018; 126(1): 74–106.

Arrow KJ. Uncertainty and the welfare economics of medical care. *American Economic Review* 1963; 53(5): 941–997.

Arrow KJ. *Essays in the Theory of Risk-Bearing*. Markham; 1971.

Barra M, Broqvist M, Gustavsson E, et al. Severity as a priority setting criterion: Setting a challenging research agenda. *Health Care Analysis* 2020; 28(1): 25–44.

Basu A, Carlson J, Veenstra D. Health years in total: A new health objective function for cost-effectiveness analysis. *Value in Health* 2020; 23(1): 96–103.

Becker GS, Phillipson TJ, Soares RR. The quantity and quality of life and the evolution of world inequality. *American Economic Review* 2005; 95(1): 277–291.

Blume-Kohout, ME, Sood N. Market size and innovation: Effects of Medicare Part D on pharmaceutical research and development. *Journal of Public Economics* 2013; 97: 327–336.

Bovenberg J, Penton H, Buyukkarmamiki N. 10 years of end-of-life criteria in the United Kingdom. *Value in Health* 2021; 24: 691–698.

Brouwer WBF, Culyer AJ, van Exel NJA, Rutten FFH. Welfarism vs. extra-welfarism. *Journal of Health Economics* 2008; 324–338.

Buckingham K, Devlin N. A theoretical framework for TTO valuations of health. *Health Economics* 2006; 15: 1149–1154.

Cameron D, Ubels J, Norström F. On what basis are medical cost-effectiveness thresholds set? Clashing opinions and an absence of data: A systematic review. *Global Health Action* 2018; 11(1): 1447828.

Chernew M, Newhouse JP. Health care spending growth. In MV Pauly, TG McGuire, P Barros, eds., *Handbook of Health Economics* (Vol. 2, pp. 1–43). North Holland; 2012.

Christensen LR, Jorgenson DW, Lau LJ. Transcendental logarithmic utility functions. *American Economic Review* 1975; 65(3): 367–383.

Claxton K, Martin S, Soares M, et al. Methods for the estimation of the National Institute for Health and Care Excellence cost-effectiveness threshold. *Health Technology Assessment* 2015; 19(4): 1–503.

Coast J. Maximisation in extra-welfarism: A critique of the current position in health economics. *Social Science & Medicine* 2009; 69: 786–792.

Cordoba JC, Ripoll M. Risk aversion and the value of life. *Review of Economic Studies* 2017; 84(4): 1472–1509.

Danzon P, Towse A, Mestre-Fernandez J. Value-based differential pricing: Efficient prices for drugs in a global context. *Health Economics* 2015; 24(3): 294–301.

Diamond PA. Cardinal welfare, individualistic ethics, and interpersonal comparison of utility: Comment. *Journal of Political Economy* 1967; 75(5): 765.

Donaldson MS, Sox HC, eds. *Setting Priorities for Health Technology Assessment: A Model Process*. National Academies Press; 1992.

Dubois P, de Mouzon O, Scott-Morton F, Seabright P. Market size and pharmaceutical innovation. *RAND Journal of Economics* 2015; 46(4): 844–871.

Easterlin RA. Explaining happiness. *Proceedings of the National Academy of Sciences of the USA* 2003; 100(19): 11176–11183.

Edwards W, Barron FH. SMARTS and SMARTER: Improved simple methods for multi-attribute utility measurement. *Organizational Behavior and Human Decision Processes* 1994; 60(3): 306–325.

Elbasha EH. Risk aversion and uncertainty in cost-effective analysis: The expected-utility, moment-generating approach. *Health Economics* 2005; 14: 457–470.

Finkelstein A. Static and dynamic effects of health policy: Evidence from the vaccine industry. *Quarterly Journal of Economics* 2004; 119(2): 527–564.

Fischhoff B, Parker AM, Bruine De Bruin W, et al. Teen expectations for significant life events. *Public Opinion Quarterly* 2000; 64(2): 189–205.

Garber AM, Phelps CE. The economic foundations of cost-effectiveness analysis. *Journal of Health Economics* 1997; 16(1): 1–31.

Gerdtham G, Jonnson B. International comparisons of health expenditures: Theory, data and econometric analysis. In AJ Culyer, JP Newhouse, eds., *Handbook of Health Economics* (Vol. 1, pp. 11–53). Elsevier; 2000.

Gloria MAJ, Thavorncharoensap M, Chaikledkawe U, Youngkong S, Thakkinstian A, Culyer AJ. A systematic review of demand-side methods of estimating the societal monetary value of health gain. *Value in Health* 2021; 243(10): 1423–1434.

Graff-Zivin J. Cost effectiveness with risk aversion. *Health Economics* 2001; 10: 499–508.

Grossman M. *The Demand for Health: A Theoretical and Empirical Investigation.* Columbia University Press (for the National Bureau for Economic Research); 1972a.

Grossman M. On the concept of health capital and the demand for health. *Journal of Political Economy* 1972b; 80(2): 223–255.

Grossman M. The human capital model. In AJ Culyer, JP Newhouse, eds., *Handbook of Health Economics*, Elsevier; 2000.

Gu Y, Lancsar E, Ghijben P, Butler JR, Donaldson C. Attributes and weights in health care priority setting: A systematic review of what counts and to what extent. *Social Sciences in Medicine* 2015; 146: 41–52.

Hanemann M. Willingness to pay and willingness to accept: How much can they differ? *American Economic Review* 1991; 81(3): 635–647.

Harsanyi J. Cardinal welfare, individualistic ethics, and interpersonal comparisons of utility. *Journal of Political Economy* 1955; 63(4): 309–321.

Hirth RA, Chernew ME, Miller E, Fendrick AM, Weissert WG. Willingness to pay for a quality-adjusted life year: In search of a standard. *Medical Decision Making* 2000; 20: 332–342.

Holt C, Laury SK. Risk aversion and incentive effects. *American Economic Review* 2002; 92(5): 1644–1655.

Horowitz JK, McConnell KE. A review of WTA/WTP studies. *Journal of Environmental Economics and Management* 2002; 44: 426–447.

Iezzoni LI, Rao SR, Bolcic-Jankovic RD, et al. Physicians' perceptions of people with disability and their health care. *Health Affairs* 2021; 40(2): 297–306.

Jonas DE, Ferrari RM, Wines RC, et al. Evaluating evidence on intermediate outcomes: Considerations for groups making healthcare recommendations. *American Journal of Preventive Medicine* 2018; 54(Suppl.): S38–S52.

Kaplan EL, Meier P. Nonparametric estimation from incomplete observations. *Journal of the American Statistical Association* 1958; 53(282): 457–481.

Keeney RL. Multiplicative utility functions. *Operations Research* 1974; 22(1): 22–34.

Kimball MS. Precautionary saving in the small and in the large. *Econometrica* 1990; 58(1): 53–73.

Kneisner TJ, Viscusi WK, Ziliak JP. Life cycle consumption and the age-adjusted value of life. *B. E. Journal of Economic Analysis & Policy* 2004; 5(1): 1–36.

Lakdawalla D, Sood, N. Health insurance as a two-part pricing contract. *Journal of Public Economics* 2013; 102: 1–12.

Lakdawalla DN. Economics of the pharmaceutical industry. *Journal of Economic Literature* 2018; 56(2): 397–449.

Lakdawalla DN, Doshi JA, Garrison LP, Phelps CE, Basu A, Danzon PM. Defining elements of value in health care—A health economics approach: An ISPOR Special Task Force report. *Value in Health* 2018; 21: 131–139.

Lakdawalla DN, Phelps CE. Health technology assessment with risk-aversion in health. *Journal of Health Economics* 2020; 72: 102346.

Lakdawalla DN, Phelps CE. Health technology assessment with diminishing returns to health: The generalized risk-adjusted cost-effectiveness (GRACE) approach. *Value in Health* 2021a; 24(2): 244–249.

Lakdawalla DN, Phelps CE. A guide to extending and implementing generalized risk-adjusted cost-effectiveness (GRACE). *European Journal of Health Economics* 2021b; 23(3): 433–451.

Law A, Pathak D, McCord M. Health utility assessment by standard gamble: A comparison of the probability equivalence and lottery equivalence approaches. *Pharmaceutical Research* 1998; 15(1): 105–109.

Lerner AP. The concept of monopoly and the measurement of monopoly power. *Review of Economic Studies* 1934; 1(3); 157–175.

Li M, Basu A, Bennette CS, Veenstra DL, Garrison LP. Do cancer treatments have option value? Real-world evidence from metastatic melanoma. *Health Economics* 2019; 28(7): 855–867.

Lichtenstein S, Slovic P, Fischhoff B, Combs B. Judged frequency of lethal events. *Journal of Experimental Psychology: Human Learning and Memory* 1978; 4: 551–578.

Linley WG, Hughes DA. Societal views on NICE, cancer drugs fund and value-based pricing criteria for prioritising medicines: A cross-sectional survey of 4118 adults in Great Britain: Societal preferences for the funding of medicines. *Health Economics* 2013; 22(8): 948–964.

Loury GC. Market structure and innovation. *Quarterly Journal of Economics* 1979; 93(3): 395–410.

Madhavan G. *Applied Minds: How Engineers Think*. Norton; 2016.

Martín-Fernández J, del Cura-González MI, Gómez-Gascón T, et al. Differences between willingness to pay and willingness to accept for visits by a family physician: A contingent valuation study. *BMC Public Health* 2010; 10: article 236.

Maynard A. Developing the healthcare market. *Economic Journal* 1991; 101(408): 1277–1286.

Meyer DJ, Meyer J. Relative risk aversion: What do we know? *Journal of Risk and Uncertainty* 2005; 31(3): 243–262.

Murphy K, Topel R. The value of health and longevity. *Journal of Political Economy* 2006; 114(5): 871–904.

National Institute for Health and Care Excellence. NICE health technology evaluations: The manual; 2022. https://www.nice.org.uk/process/pmg36/chapter/introduction-to-health-technology-evaluation

Neumann PJ, Sanders GD, Russell LB, Siegel JE, Ganiats TG. *Cost-Effectiveness in Health and Medicine* (2nd ed.). Oxford University Press; 2017.

Newhouse JP, Insurance Experiment Group. *Free for All? Lessons from the RAND Health Insurance Experiment*. Harvard University Press; 1996.

Noussair CN, Trautmann ST, Van de Kuilen G. Higher order risk attitudes, demographics, and financial decisions. *Review of Economic Studies* 2014; 81(1): 325–355.

Nord E, Pinto JL, Richardson J, Menzel P, Ubel P. Incorporating societal concerns for fairness in numerical valuations of health programmes. *Health Economics* 1999; 8(1): 25–39.

Nordhaus WD. An economic theory of technical change. *American Economic Review* 1969a; 59(2): 18–28.

Nordhaus WD. *Invention, Growth and Welfare*. MIT Press; 1969b.

Ottersen T, Førde R, Kakad M, et al. A new proposal for priority setting in Norway: Open and fair. *Health Policy* 2016; 120(3): 246–251.

Pauly MV. The questionable economic case for value-based drug pricing in market health systems. *Value Health* 2017; 20(2): 278–282.

Phelps CE. Good interventions gone bad. *Medical Decision Making* 1997; 17(1): 107–112.

Phelps CE. *Health Economics* (6th ed.). Routledge; 2018.

Phelps CE. A new method for determining the optimal willingness to pay in cost-effectiveness analysis. *Value in Health* 2019a; 22(7): 785–791.

Phelps CE. When opportunity knocks, what does it say?" *Value in Health* 2019b; 22(8): 851–853.

Phelps CE. Information diffusion and best practice adoption. In JP Newhouse, AJ Culyer, eds., *Handbook of Health Economics* (Vol. 1, pp. 223–263). Elsevier; 2000.

Phelps CE. Optimal health insurance. *Journal of Risk and Insurance*, March 21, 2022a. https://doi.org/10.1111/jori.12377

Phelps CE. *Risk aversion in the large and in the small.* Working paper, University of Rochester; 2022b.

Phelps CE, Cinatl C. Estimating optimal willingness to pay thresholds for cost-effectiveness analysis: A generalized method. *Health Economics* 2021; 30(7): 1697–1702.

Phelps CE, Lakdawalla DN. Methods to Adjust Willingness to Pay (WTP) for Severity of Illness. *Value in Health* 2023; 26(7): 1003–1010.

Phelps CE, Lakdawalla DN, Basu A, Drummond MF, Towse A, Danzon PM. Approaches to aggregation and decision making—A health economics approach: An ISPOR Special Task Force report. *Value in Health* 2018; 21: 146–154.

Phelps CE, Madhavan G. Using multi-criteria approaches to assess the value of health care. *Value in Health* 2017; 20(2): 251–255.

Phelps CE, Madhavan G. *Making Better Choices: Decisions, Design and Democracy.* New York: Oxford University Press; 2021.

Phelps CE, Mooney C. Correction and update on priority setting in medical technology assessment in medical care. *Medical Care* 1992; 31(8): 744–775.

Phelps CE, Parente ST. Priority setting in medical technology and medical practice assessment. *Medical Care* 1990; 29(8): 703–723.

Phelps CE, Parente ST. *The Economics of US Health Care Policy.* Routledge; 2017.

Phelps CE, "On the (Near) Equivalence of Welfarist and Extra-Welfarist Methods to Value Healthcare," *Value in Health*, 2023 Aug 17; doi: 10.1016/j.jval.2023.08.001.

Phelps CE, Lakdawalla DN, "Methods to Adjust Willingness-to-Pay Measures for Severity of Illness," *Value in Health*, 2023; 26(7):1003-1010. doi: 10.1016/j.jval.2023.02.001.

Philipson TJ, Jena AB. Who benefits from new medical technologies? Estimates of consumer and producer surpluses for HIV/AIDS drugs. *Forum for Health Economics & Policy* 2006; 9(2): 1–33.

Pratt JW. Risk aversion in the small and in the large. *Econometrica* 1964; 32(1): 122–136.

Ramsey FP. A contribution to the theory of taxation. *Economic Journal* 1927; 37(145): 47–61.

Rawls J. *A Theory of Justice.* Belknap; 1971.

Reckers-Droog VT, van Exel NJA, Brouwer WBF. Looking back and moving forward: On the application of proportional shortfall in healthcare priority setting in the Netherlands. *Health Policy* 2018; 122(6): 621–629.

Rosen S. The value of changes in life expectancy. *Journal of Risk and Uncertainty* 1988; 1(3): 285–304.

Rothschild M, Stiglitz J. Equilibrium in competitive insurance markets: An essay on the economics of imperfect information. *Quarterly Journal of Economics* 1976; 90(4): 630–649.

Rutten-van Mouken MPMH, Bakker CH, van Doorslaer EKA, van der Linden S. Methodological issues of patient utility measurement: Experience from two clinical trials. *Medical Care* 1995; 33(9): 922–937.

Ryen I, Svensson M. The willingness to pay for a quality adjusted life year: A review of the empirical literature. *Health Economics* 2015; 24: 1289–1301.

Saha A. Expo-power utility: A "flexible" form for absolute and relative risk aversion. *American Journal of Agricultural Economics* 1993; 75(4): 905–913.

Sanchez Y, Penrod JR, Qiu XL, Romley J, Snider JT, Phillipson T. The option value of innovative treatments in the context of chronic myeloid leukemia. *American Journal of Managed Care* 2012; 18(11 Suppl.): S265–S271.

Schosser S, Trarbach JN, Vogt B. How does the perception of pain determine the selection of different treatments? Experimental evidence for convex utility functions over pain duration and concave utility functions over pain intensity. *Journal of Economic Behavior & Organization* 2016; 131(B): 174–182.

Shah KK. Severity of illness and priority setting in healthcare: A review of the literature. *Health Policy* 2009; 93(2–3): 77–84.

Shakespeare W. *The Tragedy of King Richard the Third, circa* 1593. Printed in 1597 by Valentine Sims for Andrew Wife, dwelling in Paules Church-yard, at the Signe of the Angell.

Shiroiwa T, Igarashi A, Fukuda T, Ikeda S. WTP for a QALY and health states: More money for severer health states? *Cost Effectiveness and Resource Allocation* 2013; 11: 22.

Skedgel C, Henderson N, Towse A, Mott D. Considering severity in health technology assessment: Can we do better?" *Value in Health* 2022; 25(8): 1399–1403. https://doi.org/10.1016/j.jval.2022.02.004

Snider JT, Romley JA, Voght WB, Philipson TJ. The option value of innovation. *Forum for Health Economics & Policy* 2012; 15(2). :/j/fhep.2012.15.issue-2/1558-9544.1306/1558-9544.1306.xml

Tan-Torres Edjerer R, Baltussen T, Hutubessy A, et al. *Making Choices in Health: WHO Guide to Cost-Effectiveness Analysis*. World Health Organization; 2003.

Towse A, Barnsley P. Clarifying meanings of absolute and proportional shortfall with examples. https://www.nice.org.uk/Media/Default/About/what-we-do/NICE-guidance/NICE-technology-appraisals/OHE-Note-on-proportional-versus-absolute-shortfall.pdf. 17 September 2013.

Tunçel T, Hammitt JK. A new meta-analysis on the WTP/WTA disparity. *Journal of Environmental Economics and Management* 2014; 68: 175–187.

Vanness DJ, Lomas J, Ahn H. A health opportunity cost threshold for cost-effectiveness analysis in the United States. *Annals of Internal Medicine* 2021; 194(1): 25–32.

Verguet S, Kim JJ, Jamison DT. Extended cost-effectiveness analysis for health policy assessment: A tutorial. *Pharmacoeconomics* 2016; 34: 913–923.

Viscusi WK. *Smoking: Making the Risky Decision*. Oxford University Press; 1992.

Viscusi WK, Aldy JE. The value of a statistical life: A critical review of market estimates throughout the world. *Journal of Risk and Uncertainty* 2003; 27(1): 5–76.

Viscusi WK, Gayer T. Behavioral public choice: The behavioral paradox of government policy. *Harvard Journal of Law and Public Policy* 2015; 38: 973–1007.

Viscusi WK, Hakes J. Risk perceptions and smoking behavior. *Economic Inquiry* 2008; 48(1): 45–59.

Weibull W. A statistical distribution of wide applicability. *ASME Journal of Applied Mechanics* 1951; 18(3): 293–297.

Williams A. The economics of coronary bypass grafting. *British Medical Journal* 1985; 291: 326–329.

Williams A. Cost-effectiveness analysis: Is it ethical? *Journal of Medical Ethics* 1992; 18: 7–11.

Williams A. Intergenerational equity: An exploration of the fair innings argument. *Health Economics* 1997; 6: 117–132.

Williams A. *What could be nicer than NICE?* Office of Health Economics Annual Lecture; 2004. https://www.ohe.org/publications/what-could-be-nicer-nice

World Health Organization. *Choosing interventions That Are Cost-effective.* World Health Organization; 2014.

For the benefit of digital users, indexed terms that span two pages (e.g., 52–53) may, on occasion, appear on only one of those pages.

Tables, figures, and boxes are indicated by *t*, *f*, and *b* following the page number.